# SURVIVING
## FEELINGS

# SURVIVING
# FEELINGS

## A Manual For Overcoming Dark Emotions

Michael A. Caparrelli, Jr., PhD

# COPYPRIGHT

# CONTENTS

# FOREWORD

I consider Michael Caparrelli to be a spiritual son. We met when he visited my church as a "seeker" 26 years ago. I was part of the prayer team that met him at the altar when he received Jesus Christ as his Lord and Savior. Later, when we became more personally acquainted as co-workers and associate pastors in that same church, he would routinely casually stroll into my office, seat himself in the chair across from my desk and pose a question regarding a particular scripture or Biblical principle. Then my mind would race down a track of knowledge; searching for a satisfactory answer to his quest. Sometimes I found the finish line. Sometimes I didn't. Sometimes the discourse just created more questions. I was intrigued by his seemingly unquenchable thirst for knowledge.

Michael and I have been friends now for many years. While it is true that he is boldly brilliant and possesses a genius of multifaceted giftedness, it is the heart of the man that shines brightest in my eyes. His years of pastoring at Sacred Exchange Fellowship (Rhode Island) expanded his compassion for the bleeding and the broken as he looked towards God for answers on how to best help them. Undoubtedly, God fashioned Michael's heart to reflect His.

Michael is a very educated and learned man who knows that of which he speaks and teaches. But it isn't knowledge that sets him apart. It's his big fat heart that bleeds for the bleeding and breaks for the broken. This book is just one more effort on his part to help. It is a vast array of information coupled with experience and a sprinkling of humor to help us gain some ground in our quest for wholeness.

I personally understand the importance of this quest. By the time I was 27 years old my emotions were frozen; and although it continued to beat, my heart had flatlined and my face reflected what I felt – nothing! Childhood trauma grew into teenage trauma, which morphed into adult trauma. With every phase, I stuffed feeling after feeling until I no longer felt anything.

After years of drug addiction, institutionalization and criminal behavior, I found myself in a discipleship program known as Teen Challenge. It was there that Jesus Christ captured and melted my icy heart with the warmth of His love. Emotions began to flow (or rather flood) in all directions. Although it was good to feel alive again, I had no clue what to do with all that I was feeling.

Even with Jesus as a traveling companion, my road to emotional and mental health was a complicated, lengthy, and painful journey. I learned a lot in college as I read and studied towards a degree in Social Work. I talked with friends and spiritual leaders. I spent time in counseling and being guided by professionals. I immersed myself in countless hours of prayer and reading God's word, which really helped.

Each phase of the healing process offered me new insights and progress. I understood that the process was an active one of which I had a part to play. Of course, no matter how healthy we become, each of us is still a work in progress as Holy Spirit continues His assignment to fashion us into the beautiful and perfect image of Jesus Christ.

"And I am certain that God, who began the good work within you, will continue the work until it is finally finished on the day when Christ Jesus returns" (Philippians 1:6 NLT).

You may have heard the terms mental health and emotional health used interchangeably. However, there is a distinction. Mental health is about processing information that presents itself in everyday circumstances, while emotional health is more about processing and managing the emotions that arise because of that information. It is a type of symbiotic relationship between our hearts and our heads.

Although some folks claim not to be emotional, and they may even mock those who are as "touchy-feely", their claim is not really true. All human beings have emotions and feel things. Of course, some of us feel more deeply and are more sensitive than others. At different times in our lives we all can feel emotions like anger, fear, love, sadness, shame, anxiety, and more.

Emotions, and the fact that we feel them, are not the problem. Difficulties arise when we don't process them in a healthy and productive manner. Instead of going for a run, writing in a journal, punching a pillow, taking a shower, listening to worship music, cleaning a closet, praying, sharing with a friend, walking the dog, watching a funny movie, or eating ice cream (YES!)...we choose something less helpful. We may decide to open a bottle of beer, pop a few pills, stay in bed, stop eating, eat too much, punch a wall (or a person), throw things, curse God, stop answering our phone (or never get off our phone), vent on Facebook, stuff our feelings, or deny what is happening.

Emotions are here to stay. Understanding and managing them in a healthy way should be our goal. That's why this book is so important. It is like a "how to" read about identifying what we are feeling, understanding how it relates to us, and considering the most appropriate way to respond. Or as Dr. Mike describes the process: NAME IT, FRAME IT, and TAME IT.

Our world is plagued with poor mental health for reasons both simple and complex. I hope you won't just glance over the few statistics I am about to share. Allow the reality of the data to open your eyes to the dilemma of America's mental health crisis courtesy of the National Alliance on Mental Health.

In 2020, almost 53 million adults experienced mental health issues (1 in 5), suicide is the second leading cause of death among those aged 10-34 in the United Stated, and 70% of youth in the juvenile justice system have a diagnosed emotional/mental health condition. We are not well. We need help.

There are many who may need more than a self-help book can offer. But there are many who could become healthier by reading a book like this and applying the truth found within its pages. I don't know where you, the reader, can be found on the scale of emotional and mental health. You may have even picked up this book for a family member or friend. Either way, I applaud you!

Change will not come overnight. But if you will adhere to the truth of the Gospel and appreciate the discoveries of neuroscience, I can assure you it will come. (Additionally, if you have not yet read Dr. Mike's book entitled, "Dr. Jesus: Devotions for Your Mental Health", I urge you to get a copy.)

We are all broken people when we come to Christ. Thinking that once we become a Christian we are "all set" is a fallacy. True enough, He will lead us to a place of wholeness if we are willing to be led and remain open to instruction and guidance. But many of us stay stuck. May I encourage you to move forward on the journey so you will be better equipped to fulfill your destiny and make a positive impact on this world for Jesus?

Shalom is a Hebrew word that can just be translated as peace. But the fullest definition is peace, harmony, wholeness, completeness, prosperity, welfare, fullness, and tranquility. Quite simply: Nothing missing and nothing broken. Jesus said He left His peace with us (John 14:27). I would like to leave you with that same blessing and hope for fulfillment. This book will help you navigate such a place within your own heart and mind.

SHALOM!

Jacqui Strothoff,
Founder of Teen Challenge Providence Women's Home

# INTRODUCTION

Your brain consists of an ANALYST and an ANIMAL, two regions that God hardwired into your neurobiological makeup (See diagram below). The analyst signifies the frontal cortex - the hub of critical reasoning. Your analyst enables you to balance your checkbook, weigh the pros and cons of a decision, solve problems, fix the lawnmower and execute a multiplicity of rational functions. Without your analyst, you would make costly decisions. Your analyst is the director of your life.

The animal, on the other hand, signifies the limbic system - the center of emotional processing. Your animal empowers you to instinctually respond to a crisis, empathize with people, and a host of other emotional functions. Without your animal, you would never make it through life. Your analyst isn't swift enough to dodge an oncoming car or fight off an intruder. Only the animal can handle such high-pressure situations. Your inner animal is the protector of your life.

If you'd prefer biblical terms for these biological realities, the closest examples you'll find within the scriptures are mentioned by Jesus in Matthew 22:37. Jesus' usage of the term "mind" refers to that rational part of us (the analyst) whereas His usage of the term "heart" signifies the emotional-instinctual part of us (the animal).

Let's do a comparative review. The analyst is the logical/rational part of you whereas the animal is the emotional/instinctual part of you. The analyst guides you through everyday situations whereas the animal assists you during a crisis. The analyst is slow and calculating whereas the animal is swift and intuitive. The analyst is the director of your life whereas the animal is the protector of your life. Get it?

Now, let's talk about the animal on a deeper level because it's the region of your brain that gets you into the most trouble. The animal makes a wonderful servant but a horrible master. When the animal serves me, I instinctually respond to a crisis without dumbness or delay. But when the animal masters me, I punch walls, pop pills, sleep around, sleep late, people-please, argue too much, and fall prey to every lustful desire.

Unruly emotions are the result of the inner animal gone wild, a limbic system that's lost its cool. Let's face it; feelings such as grief, fear, and anger are an inescapable part of life. These feelings are no less frequent for the believer than for the skeptic. Read the book of Psalms and you'll see what I mean. However, it's one thing to have anger; it's another thing for anger to have you. It's one thing to have fear; it's another thing for fear to have you (Hence the reason why the Apostle Paul describes fear as a "spirit" in II Timothy 1:7 rather than just a feeling to connote the kind of fear that has a grip on you). Unmanageable feelings are the result of your inner animal losing control.

Here's another way of looking at the uncontrollable animal, a.k.a. the overly emotional mind. The animal region of your brain hosts your four survival instincts - fight, flight, freeze, and fawn. The fighting instinct helps you to defend yourself or the people you love from intruders. The flight instinct enables you to circumvent life-threatening situations. The freeze instinct causes you to remain still when movement would be detrimental. The fawn instinct equips you with the wisdom to empathize with your opponents, appease their wrath and even negotiate out of dangerous situations. If you've ever heard the true story of the Cleveland woman held hostage by her looney captor for many years, you've encountered a woman with good fawn instincts to survive that long.

When your animal is out of control, your survival instincts backfire on you. You're too aggressive - you fight with people there's no reason to fight with. You're too avoidant - you flight from settings such as a church, the workplace, or even a marriage at the sight of any offense. You're too ambivalent - you freeze at every decision point. You're too appeasing - you fawn with your opponents to the point of people-pleasing and moral compromise. Being overly aggressive, avoidant, ambivalent, and appeasing is the story of those with an unruly animal.

All of this begs the question, how do you tame an unruly animal? In other words, how do you control your unruly emotions? If you don't learn to tame that animal, you'll get yourself into trouble. The beast in you will eventually devour the best of you. Look back at your life. Take into account all of the moments when your unmanaged feelings nearly sabotaged your life. Think about all of the reckless decisions you made when you were afraid. Reflect upon all of the foolish choices when you were depressed or stressed. Untamed emotions are the reason why prisons are overcrowded with murderers and hospitals are crammed with patients.

Managing unruly emotions require three remedies - emotional identification ("name it"), emotional validation ("frame it") and emotional regulation ("tame it"). Any good therapist will offer these remedies within their sessions. This book, "Surviving Feelings", is a devotional that helps you name, frame, and tame every intense feeling that overtakes you. Again, if you don't manage that unruly animal, the beast in you will devour the best of you. Your feelings without any restraint sabotage your life.

Emotional identification, also known as "naming it", consists of identifying the specific feeling that plagues you. Too often, we have no grasp of what we feel. Think about how a dog-whisperer establishes a bond with the ferocious canine. The rapport begins by whispering the dog's name. You have no leverage over something if you don't know its name. A study performed by UCLA professor Matthew D. Lieberman indicated that naming your specific feelings alleviates their intensity. For instance, when an angry feeling is named for what it is - "I feel frustrated" - Lieberman and researchers observed a decreased response in the amygdala (the animal) and heightened activity in the ventrolateral prefrontal cortex (the analyst). A mood inventory is provided to help you name what you feel.

Emotional validation, also known as "framing it", consists of providing your feeling with a bordering context. This devotional offers you a handful of bible passages that relate to feelings. Within these passages, you'll encounter men and women who conveyed those same feelings you're experiencing. These references validate your emotions rather than dismiss them as phantoms. Your struggle is real, my friends, as there are many witnesses before you who experienced those same emotions. The provided passages will provide a framework that validates your emotions as a bona fide experience.

Emotional regulation, also known as "taming it", involves the cerebral task of countering your feelings with facts. Scriptural truths mixed with the latest science relevant to your emotional state help you to cool down when you're at the point of blowing up. Emotional regulation means exercising dominance over your feelings with life-saving truths. Such action will NOT prevent you from having feelings but it will prohibit the feeling from having you.

The greatest struggle of life is not what you go through - a bitter divorce, a devastating betrayal, a sudden job loss, a debilitating accident, etc. The real battle is grappling with what goes through you - fear, grief, anger, confusion, etc. "Surviving Feelings" is a biblically inspired, scientifically verified, manual on how to overcome a myriad of dark emotional states. With the help of God via the usage of this book, you will survive feelings that might have otherwise destroyed you. From this moment forward, may you learn to walk your animal rather than your animal walking you.

Dr. Michael A. Caparrelli

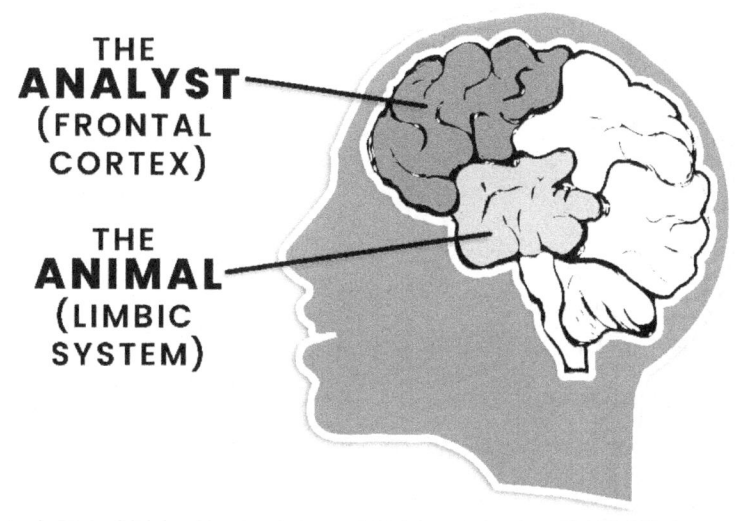

# HOW TO USE THE WORKSHEET

This is a biblically based tool designed to help you survive a difficult feeling and/or mood. With prayer and meditation, walk through the following steps anytime you are under the spell of a dark emotion. Reference the mood inventory, featured immediately after this page, to complete these steps on the worksheet after every "I Feel…" devotional.

Name the Feeling (Identification)

Identify your primary emotion – Anger, Sadness, Fear or Emptiness. Then, identify your secondary emotion which is a derivative of the primary emotion. Secondary emotions are listed under each primary emotion. Admit to God, yourself and another trusted person, "I'm feeling jealous" or "I'm feeling hopeless", or whatever emotion plagues you. Write down what you feel. Remember, feelings aren't right or wrong. They just are.

Frame the Feeling (Validation)

Select a scripture listed at the bottom of your emotional column (Anger, Sadness, etc) from the first grouping of scriptures. The first grouping consists of passages about others who have felt what you feel. In fact, even great men and women of God have experienced that same emotion. You are not alone in what you feel. The struggle is not fictitious but real. Write down how you relate to the person or persons featured in that selected scripture. You are in good company, my friend.

Tame the Feeling (Regulation)

Select a scripture listed at the bottom of your emotional column from the second grouping of scriptures. The second grouping consists of passages that appeal to our analyst, empowering our head to rule over our heart. It's okay to have an emotion, but don't let that emotion have you. It's time to tame that wild animal and keep it from mastering you. Write down any thoughts you have about the verse you selected as well as the "I Feel…" devotional and how you will apply it today.

# MOOD INVENTORY CHART

| ANGER | SADNESS | FEAR | EMPTINESS |
|---|---|---|---|
| Annoyed | Crushed | Panicky | Bored |
| Livid | Mournful | Paralyzed | Tempted |
| Frustrated | Despairing | Doubtful | Aimless |
| Disobedient | Heavy | Insecure | Blank |
| Disgusted | Lonely | Suspicious | Detached |
| Frustrated | Hurt | Worried | Apathetic |
| Resentful / Bitter | Disappointed | Hyper-vigilant | Dry |
| Offended | Hopeless | Terrified | Tired |
| Jealous | Sensitive | Shocked | Weak |
| Ex. 32:19, Jer. 15:17, Judges 14:19, Neh. 4:11, Ps. 3, 40, 69, 109, 137, Jonah 4:1, Matt. 21:12-17, Acts 17:16.<br><br>Gen. 4:5-6, 49:7, Eccl. 7:9, Prov. 14:17, 15:18, 29:22, Matt. 5:21-23, Gal. 5:22, Eph. 4:26-31, James 1:19-20, Col. 3:8. | Gen. 6:6, 23:2, 37:34-36, Judges 11:37, Ps. 44, 60, 74, 79, 80, 85, 90, Lamentations, Luke 22:62, John 11:35.<br><br>2 Sam. 12:20, Ps 3:3, 30:5,11, Isaiah 30:19, 61:3, Nehemiah 8:10, Matt. 5:4, Luke 9:60, 1 Thes. 4:13-14, Rev. 5:5, 21:4. | Gen. 3:10, 20:11, 2 Sam. 6:9, Ps. 3, Mark 4:35-41, 14:33, Luke 22:54-62, 24:37, 1 Cor. 2:3, 2 Cor. 4:8-9, Heb. 12:21.<br><br>Joshua 1:9, Ps. 23, 46, Prov. 27:1, 29:25, 31:21, Isaiah 43:1-2, Jer. 1:8, Luke 5:10, John 14:27, Acts 18:9, Phil. 4:6-7, Heb. 13:5, 2 Tim. 1:7, 1 John 4:18. | Gen. 8:22, 25:30, Judges 15:19, Num. 20:2, Eccl., Ps. 37:2, Proverbs 30:16, Isaiah 1:30, 24:3-23, Ezek. 19:13, Matt. 4:1-11, John 4:6.<br><br>Ps. 1:3, 68:6, 81:10, 107:35, Ezek. 36:26, Isaiah 40:4, 58:11, Matt. 5:6, 11:28-30, Luke 3:5, 11:24, Eph. 3:17-19. |

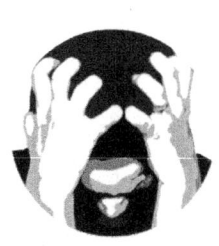

# I FEEL LIKE I'M GONNA EXPLODE

*Instead, his delight is in the Lord's instruction, and he meditates on it day and night.*

Psalm 1:1

"I don't know how to meditate", folks mistakenly presume. The facts are, if you know how to ruminate, you know how to meditate. Rumination is the practice of cognitively rehashing over and over something bothersome - an insult from your spouse, a lack of appreciation from your employer, etc. Meditation works the same way. When you meditate, you rehearse something repeatedly within your mind. I'll bet my bottom dollar you ruminated over irksome data for at least 15 minutes yesterday. "I can't believe he said that to me. Where does he get the nerve to treat me that way?" If you know how to ruminate, you know how to meditate!

While rumination and meditation share a similar modus operandi, the outcomes are vastly different. Rumination almost always leads to conniptions. For instance, while driving home yesterday, you repeatedly review what your wife spewed before you left. By the time you pull into the driveway, you're ready to explode. One wrong glance from the gal and you'll blow your lid. Conversely, meditation produces, not conniptions, but composure. Neurological studies using an EEG show that meditation activates frontal lobe regions that control our impulses. What's truly amazing is that these effects on impulse control continue for hours after the practice of meditation (Korponay, 2019).

How you meditate isn't nearly as paramount as what you meditate on. Knowing how to chew is one thing; knowing what to chew on is a much more essential subject. Chew on tobacco and watch your health deteriorate. Chew on something nutritious and watch your body revitalize. The Psalmist encourages us to chew on the word of God; a soul vitamin that restores our cells and sedates every wild impulse.

The General Movement Assessment (Frontiers in Psychology, Einspieler, 2016)
Childhood Trauma and Maladaptive Daydreaming (Trauma Dissociation, Somer et al., 2021)

# SURVIVING FEELINGS WORKSHEET

## 1. Name it (Identification)

_____
_____
_____
_____
_____
_____
_____
_____
_____

## 2. Frame it (Validation)

_____
_____
_____
_____
_____
_____
_____
_____

## 3. Tame it (Regulation)

_____
_____
_____
_____
_____
_____
_____
_____
_____

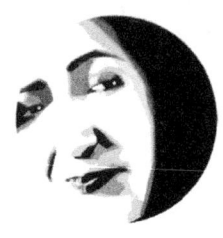

# I FEEL DESIROUS OF MONEY

*The love of money is a root of many evils.*

I Timothy 6:10

My papa would say, "money makes people funny". How tenable is this cliché? Ponder just a few of many findings from behavioral science research about the rendezvous between man and his money.

## A Decrease in Prosocial Behavior

Seven studies were performed within San Francisco where drivers are mandated to stop for pedestrians. The results indicated that drivers of luxury cars were four times less likely to let pedestrians cross than drivers of inexpensive cars (UC Berkeley, Piff, 2012).

## A Cloud over Moral Judgment

Harvard University and the University of Utah both conducted experiments on the influence of money on ethical behaviors. Results indicated that merely being exposed to money-related subjects was causative of lying and cheating (Smith-Crowe, 2013).

## A Decrease in Empathy

The University of California surveyed more than 300 upper- and lower-class participants. Respondents were asked to analyze the facial expressions of people in photos to discern their emotions. Upper-class people exhibited far less empathy than the lower class (Kraus, 2015).

Long before science warned us about money, the Bible offered 140 caveats within the Old and New Testaments. The most memorable caveat, I Timothy 6:10, puts the danger in proper perspective. Note that money itself is morally neutral; it's the "LOVE of money" that proves hazardous. The term LOVE derives from the Greek word, Philos, which means "brotherly love". God designed this affection to be reserved for Himself and fellow mankind only. Beware when you shift from using money and loving people to using people and loving money.

How The Rich Are Different From The Poor (UC Berkeley Psychology, Piff, 2012),
Organizational Behavior / Human Decision Processes (Boston University, Smith-Crowe, 2013)

# SURVIVING FEELINGS WORKSHEET

## 1. Name it (Identification)

_____

_____

_____

_____

_____

_____

_____

_____

_____

_____

## 2. Frame it (Validation)

_____

_____

_____

_____

_____

_____

_____

_____

_____

_____

## 3. Tame it (Regulation)

_____

_____

_____

_____

_____

_____

_____

_____

_____

_____

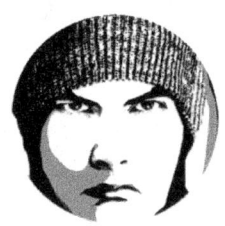

# I FEEL JUDGMENTAL

*You, therefore, have no excuse, who pass judgment on someone else, for at whatever point you judge the other, you are condemning yourself, because you do the same things. Now we know that Gods judgment is based on truth.*

Romans 2:1-2

The problem with my eyes is that I notice everyone else without seeing myself. The fact that my eyes position outward rather than inward puts me at risk for double standards. A double standard is when I'm studious of your defects but oblivious to my own, thereby condemning what you do while condoning the same defects with me. To borrow my friend Bishop Jeffery A. Williams' phrase, I got a PhD in your issues but I'm stuck in kindergarten when it comes to my own. By virtue of my facial structure alone (add to that, my massive ego), I'm prone to double standards.

The sophisticated term for Double-Standards is the Fundamental Attribution Error (FAE). FAE asserts that there are two attributions we make when explaining bad behavior - situational attributions and dispositional attributions. A situational attribution is when we blame the situation for why we acted like a Momma-Luke (Italian slang for "fool"); e.g. "I acted like a Momma-Muke because I hadn't eaten all day". A dispositional attribution is when we blame our character for why behaved stupidly; e.g. "I acted like a Momma-Luke because I am a Momma-Luke". FEA further asserts that we humans are prone to making situational attributions about our stupidity but dispositional attributions about others' foolishness. If you act like a jerk, it's because you're a jerk. But if I act like a jerk, well, let's just chalk it up as me being tired, hungry, and stressed.

The Apostle Paul rebukes such double standards in Romans 2:1. But notice what he mentions in Romans 2:2 - God's perfect judgment. Unlike our slanted perspective, God's eyes notice everything. If you want a sober assessment of yourself, don't look through your own outwardly focused eyes. That'll merely lend itself to social comparisons that puff you up. Instead, peer through God's eyes. From that vantage point, the truth will bring you to your knees rather than hoist you to a high horse.

# SURVIVING FEELINGS WORKSHEET

## 1. Name it (Identification)

_____
_____
_____
_____
_____
_____
_____
_____
_____
_____

## 2. Frame it (Validation)

_____
_____
_____
_____
_____
_____
_____
_____
_____
_____

## 3. Tame it (Regulation)

_____
_____
_____
_____
_____
_____
_____
_____
_____
_____

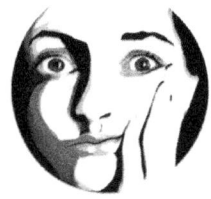

# I FEEL DRAWN TO WHAT'S FAMILIAR

*Regard not them that have familiar spirits.*

Leviticus 19:31

Demons know that humans are suckers for what's familiar. You meet someone with the same alma mater, or perhaps they smirk like your deceased father, or they hum a tune you loved as a child ...instantly, a premature trust is established. In some cases, you just made a fatal mistake by building a bond with someone on the shallow grounds of familiarity. Studies show that a car accident is more probable within a short distance from our homes than when driving in a foreign town. Why? Because at the sight and sound of what's familiar, we let our guard down. The devil, being a master strategist, is more likely to employ something familiar rather than foreign to destroy you.

A recent experiment accentuated our idiotic vulnerability to the familiar (Newman and colleagues, 2014). Participants were more likely to believe the erroneous claim, "Turtles are deaf" when it was stated by a person with a familiar name such as "Adrian" than when it was uttered by a "Czeslaw". We blindly trust whomever we can easily relate to. The first task of every conman is to establish common ground with you. "You went to Fenway Park as a kid too!", or something along these lines, is the bait that catches the fish.

Regarding Leviticus 19:31, a familiar spirit is a demon disguising itself as a dead relative. Of course, we're all suckers for our deceased relatives. Who doesn't want to chitchat with their long-dead, beloved nonna or papa? Man, I miss their stories! In a wider sense, this moniker applies to any familiar means that Satan uses to lure us into a trap. Beware - Leviticus warns us that Satan's best disguises are often pulled out of the attics of our childhood homes.

---

People With Easier To Pronounce Names Promote Truthiness of Claims (Plos One, Newman, 2014)

# SURVIVING FEELINGS WORKSHEET

## 1. Name it (Identification)

_____

_____

_____

_____

_____

_____

_____

_____

_____

_____

## 2. Frame it (Validation)

_____

_____

_____

_____

_____

_____

_____

_____

_____

## 3. Tame it (Regulation)

_____

_____

_____

_____

_____

_____

_____

_____

_____

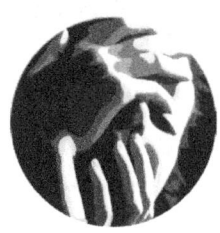

# I FEEL UNSTABLE

*"No," Jacob said, "I will continue to mourn until I join my son in the grave."*
*So his father wept for him.*
Genesis 37:35

The ups and downs of an economy are often set off by false reports. If enough rumors are spread about the stock market's dismal future, the economy nosedives into a gutter. The crash of 1929 taught us about rumors having equally as much influence over outcomes as realities. Think about it this way. How much of your anxiety or depression is set off by buying into false reports? You work yourself into a frenzy, fully persuaded you're gonna die because of a rash on your left pinky toe. You fall under a melancholy spell, entirely convinced your kids to hate you because they haven't replied to your text in the last 37 minutes.

Arbitrary Inference is a psychological theory that asserts our moods are largely affected by forming tragic conclusions without sufficient evidence. Dr. Aaron Beck (2003) observed that anxious and depressed patients possess a habit of guessing the worse possible scenarios from the slightest details. After several experiments, Beck concluded that the ups and downs of emotions are sparked by such distorted conclusions. Conversely, emotionally stable people carefully weigh the substance of a report before accepting it as legitimate.

In Genesis 37, Jacob expectedly mourns the death of his son Joseph; a despondency that prevails for years upon years. Only one problem - it's fake news! His son is not dead. Imagine, he lost years of his existence mourning over a rumor rather than a reality. If you're feeling anxious or depressed today, here are two questions to ponder. First, what conclusions am I making about the future? Second, what's the evidence to support such conclusions? Public Enemy said it right, "Don't believe the hype".

---

The Beck Depression Inventory (Beck, 2003)

# SURVIVING FEELINGS WORKSHEET

## 1. Name it (Identification)

_____

_____

_____

_____

_____

_____

_____

_____

_____

_____

_____

## 2. Frame it (Validation)

_____

_____

_____

_____

_____

_____

_____

_____

_____

_____

_____

## 3. Tame it (Regulation)

_____

_____

_____

_____

_____

_____

_____

_____

_____

_____

_____

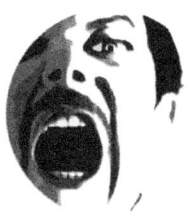

# I FEEL LIKE I WANT PAYBACK

*Do not be overcome by evil but overcome evil with good.*

Romans 12:12

A passenger was obnoxious to an airline clerk while she simply replied with a cordial smile. After the interaction, another clerk inquired, "How did you handle that jackass with such congeniality?" The clerk responded, "He's on his way to Chicago while his luggage is on its way to Des Moines". Not all avengers bite your head off but some poke at you. Revenge includes not only annihilating but irritating an enemy. "Tit for Tat" is an idiom that means an exchange of light jabs between two opponents. "Tit for Tat" avengers suppose that a light jab will satiate their anger towards an adversary while preserving their integrity (since a light jab isn't that evil).

"Tit for Tat" hardly ever works out well. First, a light jab typically provokes a reciprocal punch. As Michael Corleone told Vincent in Godfather 3 after Vincent sent Joey Zaza an ominous message, "Now Joey Zaza's gonna send you a message back." Light jabs turn petty feuds into bloody wars. Second, tit for tat is not as cathartic as avengers suppose. Colgate University performed an experiment that showed punishers brood more about an offense than non-punishers. The experiment showed that participants who engaged in "tit for tat" couldn't stop ruminating over the wrongs done to them after acts of vengeance while those who forgave moved forward without thinking much about it (Carlsmith, 2008). Revenge might be sweet initially but results in soul decay eventually.

The Apostle Paul employs a broad term for evil in Romans 12 that means "all kinds of malice". The term, malice, is not exclusive to heavy handiness but includes underhandedness. The apostle warns about being "overcome" by evil when engaging in aggressive or passive-aggressive payback plans. The term "overcome" means to be prevailed upon by an enemy. "Tit for tat" doesn't equal the score but ends the game in your demise. Only acts of goodness give you the upper hand. Instead of tit for tat, try mercy for malice.

---

The Paradoxical Consequences of Revenge (Journal of Personality and Social Psychology, Carlsmith, 2008)

# SURVIVING FEELINGS WORKSHEET

1. Name it (Identification)

_____
_____
_____
_____
_____
_____
_____
_____
_____
_____

2. Frame it (Validation)

_____
_____
_____
_____
_____
_____
_____
_____
_____
_____

3. Tame it (Regulation)

_____
_____
_____
_____
_____
_____
_____
_____
_____
_____

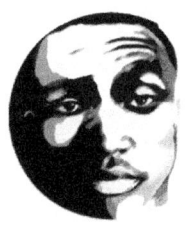

# I FEEL IMPATIENT

*He said, "Everyone brings out the choice wine first...but you have saved the best till now."*
John 2:10

Back in the 80s, we waited longer for ketchup to disperse from its glass bottle. Tip the dispenser upside down, 'shake it up baby' and your ketchup moved slower than lava. A full release took 25 seconds (10 times longer than today's squeeze bottles!), and sometimes required a knife, to slap that paste on your burger. You didn't want it to come out fast; that meant the ketchup was too thin, outdated, and vinegary. What made the wait worthwhile was knowing that a slow-release meant a thicker paste, and a thicker paste meant a high-quality delicacy. Good things come to those who wait.

A recent case study indicated that McDonald's patrons grew agitated when waiting longer than 60 seconds for their meal in line. But, once they were told that Quarter Pounders were being "made to order", Patrons became as relaxed as Jamaicans at the seaside. The case study introduced "the patience effect" which asserts that our forbearance heightens when we've been assured of receiving a better outcome for the wait.

Jesus' spectacle at the wedding of Cana didn't happen suddenly but subtlety. Instead of snapping His fingers, the Savior rolls up his sleeves. Mary & the Master of the ceremony were probably both getting crabby while waiting for Jesus' miracle. Tension permeated the air as guests were agitated by their empty glasses. No wine at a wedding was perceived as a lack of hospitality. And anytime folks feel like they're not being attended to (a.k.a., inhospitality), their feet start tapping. When the miracle finally occurs, the master of ceremony notes the reason for the delay. He saved the best for last! If your patience is wearing thin, remind yourself that a slow-release means a thicker paste. God is saving the best for last.

---

The Neuroscience of Patience (Psychology Today, Bergland, 2018)

# SURVIVING FEELINGS WORKSHEET

1. Name it (Identification)

_____

_____

_____

_____

_____

_____

_____

_____

_____

_____

2. Frame it (Validation)

_____

_____

_____

_____

_____

_____

_____

_____

_____

_____

3. Tame it (Regulation)

_____

_____

_____

_____

_____

_____

_____

_____

_____

_____

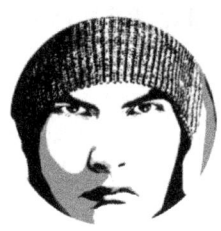

# I FEEL UPSET WITH GOD

*But a hireling - he who is not the shepherd - sees the wolf coming and leaves the sheep.... The hireling flees because he is a hireling and does not care about the sheep.*

John 10:12-13

A 7-year-old girl was sexually assaulted by her Caucasian godfather but later reported that it was an African-American stranger who violated her. Years later, after undergoing therapy, she recalled it was her godfather who committed the atrocity. She blamed an African-American stranger because she stared at a Jimmy Hendrix poster while the crime occurred. Her mind played a trick on her. The error confirmed a theory about our recollections being notoriously unreliable. Memory is not like a tape recorder that accurately plays back prior moments. Instead, memory is more like a Wikipedia page that can be revised to state something true or false.

According to Source Confusion Theory, it's easy to misattribute the source of our pain when remembering it. Since emotional memory (the feelings) and episodic memory (the facts) are stored in two different regions of the brain - emotional memory within the amygdala and episodic memory within the hippocampus - mismatching our pain with the wrong perpetrator is probable. For instance, many adults are incensed with one parent when their injuries were committed by the other parent. Since I saw mom's face (or Dad's face) every day, I hold her liable for my injuries even though she's the one who bandaged my wounds.

Indisputably, the greatest source of confusion is when we hold God responsible for the devil's villainy. Undeniably, this lie is the most fatal because it inhibits us from taking hold of the only reliable raft (the Savior) when the ocean waves engulf us. Jesus knew all about our deception-proneness; hence, the reason He contrasts the Hireling and the Shepherd in John 10. Jesus offers a key to discerning between your protector and your perpetrator - whereas your protector looked out for you, your perpetrator only looked out for themselves. Make sure you are angry with the right person.

# SURVIVING FEELINGS WORKSHEET

## 1. Name it (Identification)

_____
_____
_____
_____
_____
_____
_____
_____
_____
_____
_____

## 2. Frame it (Validation)

_____
_____
_____
_____
_____
_____
_____
_____
_____
_____

## 3. Tame it (Regulation)

_____
_____
_____
_____
_____
_____
_____
_____
_____
_____

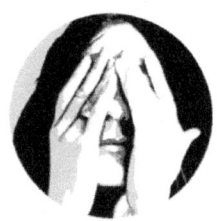

# I FEEL OBSESSED

*"In Him, all things are held together. Christ is the head of the body."*
Colossians 1:17-18

Pres. Jimmy Carter was overwhelmed with minutia by his 2nd year without a Chief of Staff. Dick Cheney warned Carter that the presidency was unfeasible without appointing such a gatekeeper. The Chief of Staff's job is to ensure that ONLY essential matters reach the president's desk, filtering everything else out. Like Carter, Obsessive-Compulsive Disorder (OCD)sufferers are flooded with minutia - a bombardment of petty details that make life an uneasy voyage. Sanitize your hands, alphabetize the canned goods, symmetrize the rug tassels, and other trivial data floods OCD sufferers' minds. Like Carter's administration, the OCD brain lacks a gatekeeper to filter out the petty stuff.

What's wrong with the OCD brain? The Basal Ganglia (a brain function) helps the psyche sort through insignificant sensory input before it reaches the conscious mind. The Basal Ganglia ensures that your mind is not flooded with minutia so that you can focus on what's essential. MRIs reveal that OCD sufferers have a "leaky filter" within the Basal Ganglia whereby neurons that enable it to execute its job ooze out. OCD sufferers are overrun by trivial details because they lack an operable Basal Ganglia, the figurative Chief of Staff who clears their minds from petty stuff.

In Colossians, Christ is depicted as "the head who holds all things together". Being a born-again believer, Christ is alive inside of you. If your head isn't working properly, you've received a new head that keeps everything in balance. For those born-again believers with a "leaky filter", trust your Savior to hold your world together. He is not only the Commander in Chief but also the Gatekeeper who preserves your sound mind.

# SURVIVING FEELINGS WORKSHEET

## 1. Name it (Identification)

_____
_____
_____
_____
_____
_____
_____
_____
_____

## 2. Frame it (Validation)

_____
_____
_____
_____
_____
_____
_____
_____
_____

## 3. Tame it (Regulation)

_____
_____
_____
_____
_____
_____
_____
_____
_____

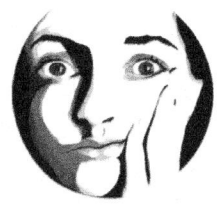

# I FEEL WORRIED

*But the Helper, the Holy Spirit, whom the Father will send in my name, he will teach you*
*all things and bring to your remembrance all things pertaining to me.*

John 14:26

If I vocalized a list of items to purchase at the supermarket, you'd most likely remember the last 2-to to 3 words on the list. I've done the exercise many times with my students in psych class, and it's nearly always the same outcome. The Recency Effect is a cognitive bias whereby our perspective of reality is defined by what's most recent. Even if a particular item is vocalized several times on that shopping list - 'bananas, bananas, bananas' - its memory is easily overwritten by what's most contemporary. Our short-term memory capacity is scant, only accommodating the latest info.

How does this psychological phenomenon affect your life? Your most recent conflict with your BFF could easily warp your perspective of the entire relationship. Don't allow this one bad moment to erase all prior moments. Your most recent blunder within the workplace could easily warp your self-image. Don't permit this one mistake to override all previous successes. And, your most recent worries at the gas pump could easily cause you to forget all of the penniless moments that God provided.

According to John 14, the Holy Spirit's role is to "bring remembrance" of Jesus. Since we possess a built-in forgetter, God assists the Born-again believer by invoking recollections of the Savior. If you're worried about the future, let the Holy Spirit remind you about the past. Not for one single moment were you ever forsaken. Don't just see the recent problems before but remember the provisions behind you.

# SURVIVING FEELINGS WORKSHEET

## 1. Name it (Identification)

_____

_____

_____

_____

_____

_____

_____

_____

_____

## 2. Frame it (Validation)

_____

_____

_____

_____

_____

_____

_____

_____

_____

## 3. Tame it (Regulation)

_____

_____

_____

_____

_____

_____

_____

_____

_____

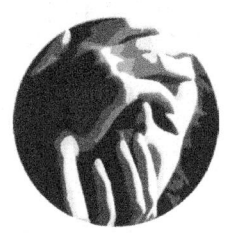

# I FEEL OVERWHELMED

*Jesus said, (after calming the storm), "Why are you so afraid? Do you still have no faith?"*
*They were terrified and asked each other, "Who is this? Even the wind and the waves obey him!"*

Mark 4:40-41

Emotions make wonderful slaves but deplorable masters. When emotions serve me, I preach passionate sermons that stir listeners' hearts. When emotions serve me, I counsel constituents with helpful empathy. When emotions serve me, I feel what must be felt without drinking or drugging. But, when emotions master me, I punch walls, eat too much cheesecake, wallow in pity, and fall prey to every vice. Emotions make faithful friends or fatal foes, ambitious servants, or vicious tyrants.

Emotions are more influential than cognitions (thoughts). The University of Massachusetts conducted a study amongst 20,000 participants that revealed emotionally-based attitudes are more prevailing than logical views. Participants read two books about aquatic animals - the first included encyclopedic facts whereas the second entailed a highly emotive experience between a swimmer and an underwater animal. After a long period, participants were surveyed on their views about these animals. Participants who read about the emotive experiences were more likely to hold their initial views about the aquatic animals than those who read encyclopedic facts. Feelings are much stickier than facts.

Within our passage of study, the real storm is not what happens to the disciples but what happens through the disciples. Peter, James, and John are petrified even after the waves are calmed. Thankfully, Jesus speaks to their souls after speaking to the storm. Now, notice what happens to their emotions after Jesus exhorts them. Their emotions aren't ejected but redirected. Jesus' words shift the disciples from being terror-stricken by the storm to being awe-struck by the Savior. Awe is a much more useful feeling than fear. When Jesus speaks to you today in church, your feelings shift from being vicious tyrants to helpful servants.

---

Attitudes Based on Feelings, Emotions Can Stand Test of Time (Sage Journals, Rocklage, 2021)

# SURVIVING FEELINGS WORKSHEET

## 1. Name it (Identification)

_____
_____
_____
_____
_____
_____
_____
_____
_____
_____

## 2. Frame it (Validation)

_____
_____
_____
_____
_____
_____
_____
_____
_____

## 3. Tame it (Regulation)

_____
_____
_____
_____
_____
_____
_____
_____
_____

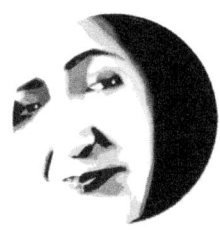

# I FEEL LIKE BLAMING SOMEONE

*Jesus said, "A man was traveling on the road to Jericho when he fell among robbers*
*who stripped him, beat him, and left him half dead."*

Luke 10:30

Almost guaranteed that if you get a flat tire while coasting with friends, someone's bound to ask, "Well, didn't you check the air pressure before we left?" Whenever something goes wrong, the human tendency is to locate a culprit. Despite Solomon's statement, "time and chance happen to all people", meaning that flat tires happen to anyone at any time, humans still hunt for a perpetrator when bad outcomes unfold. Why is the blame game so easy for us?

"Just World Fallacy" is a cognitive distortion whereby we suppose that if something bad happens to Jane, she must have done something bad. The bias is dubbed "Just World" because it's predicated upon the fallacy of a morally equitable universe that pays you what you deserve. Most claim they don't reason this way but our talk suggests otherwise - "What goes around comes around", "Karma is a $&#*", etc. The University of Illinois conducted a study that revealed a possible reason why the blame game is our default setting. The study showed a correlation between participants' belief in a "just world" and their lack of willingness to help someone in a crisis (Begue, 2008). Could it be that blaming someone for their problems justifies our unwillingness to help? "Since you didn't check the air pressure before we left, don't expect me to soil my shirt by unscrewing lug-nuts. You're on your own, pal!"

In Luke 10, Jesus sets his story on the "Road to Jericho." According to Bible commentator William Barclay, Jews believed that you were a fool if you traversed this dangerous road alone without a caravan. Highly likely is the possibility that the Levite and Priest who offered no helping hand reasoned this way about the lonesome traveler - "you are suffering the fate of fools". Maybe this is why Jesus makes it clear that the crime happened on the "road to Jericho" to offer insight into their rationale. In this case, blame is a cover-up for the unwillingness to be inconvenienced. Hidden behind the blame game is often an unwillingness to dirty our hands from changing a flat tire.

Altruistic Behavior and the Bio-dimensional Just World Belief (The American Journal of Psychology, Begue, 2008)

# SURVIVING FEELINGS WORKSHEET

## 1. Name it (Identification)

_____
_____
_____
_____
_____
_____
_____
_____
_____
_____

## 2. Frame it (Validation)

_____
_____
_____
_____
_____
_____
_____
_____
_____

## 3. Tame it (Regulation)

_____
_____
_____
_____
_____
_____
_____
_____
_____

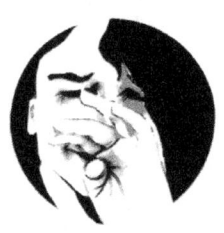

# I FEEL LONELY

*...Instead, I call you friends for everything that I learned from my Father I made known to you. John 15:15*

If I ingest vitamins as a supplement to vegetables, I'll be happy with its health results. If vitamins are my only source of nutrition, I'll foolishly curse vitamins for not doing me right. Such is the scenario with Facebook friendships. The University of Missouri conducted 4 studies that revealed when people use Facebook as a supplement for real-world friendships, they feel fulfilled from social media interactions. However, when people look to FB as a substitute for real-world friendships, loneliness skyrockets (Sheldon, 2011). FB makes a wonderful supplement, a horrible substitute.

Why are Facebook friendships a poor substitute for real-world confidants? Stony Brook University performed studies that uncovered a factor that establishes bonds - the sharing of secrets (Aaron, 1997). When I share with you my hurt feelings about a feud with dad, you feel special that I divulged such details to you alone. A bond is built at the point where classified information is exchanged. The bond deepens as reciprocity occurs. True intimacy happens when both parties say look "Into-Me-See". Facebook is a public platform where I post my opinions to anyone and everyone rather than a special someone. The platform lacks the secrecy component that makes friendships sacred.

In John 15, Jesus doesn't christen his disciples as "friends" immediately but only after investing significant time in their presence (3 years). Jesus knew the difference between a constituent and a confidant. Also, pay attention to what confirms the bond  - the sharing of secrets. He says they are friends because He's made known to them exclusive information. What Jesus says and does in the gospels is what He's saying and doing today. An invitation for friendship still stands to anyone who surrenders to Him as Lord. May I submit to you that all friendships - Facebook and the real world - are merely supplements of our bond with God? If you don't know Him, you won't feel close to anyone. Marvin Gaye said it right, "Ain't nothing like the real thing, baby".

The Experimental Generation of Interpersonal Closeness (Personality and Social Psychology, Aaron, 1997), A Two-process View of Facebook Use and Related Need-Satisfaction (Personality and Social Psychology, Sheldon, 2011)

# SURVIVING FEELINGS WORKSHEET

## 1. Name it (Identification)

_____
_____
_____
_____
_____
_____
_____
_____
_____
_____

## 2. Frame it (Validation)

_____
_____
_____
_____
_____
_____
_____
_____
_____
_____

## 3. Tame it (Regulation)

_____
_____
_____
_____
_____
_____
_____
_____
_____
_____

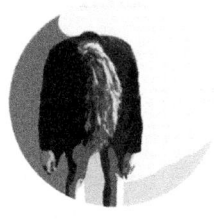

# I FEEL LAZY

*Laziness brings a deep sleep.*

Proverbs 19:5

Let your car idle for 10 minutes on a cold day and it'll be all warmed up for you. Permit your car to idle for hours and it'll run out of gas. The same is true for us. Idleness is beneficial when it occurs for brief intervals between commutes. Too much idleness results in depletion. We function best with brief, intermittent periods of rest. We function horribly when rest (not the attitude but the activity) is ongoing. In Genesis 2, God rests on the seventh day; the rest occurs for 1 day between pioneering the world (Genesis 1) and managing what He pioneered (Genesis 3). Rest was designed to repair us from yesterday's work, and restore us for tomorrow's endeavors.

Inordinate amounts of idleness negatively affect us for two reasons. First, neurotransmitters such as adrenaline and endorphins rely upon physical movement for their release. Without these energy-boosting neurotransmitters, we're prone to fall into a spell of melancholy. Second, an idle mind is prone to worry about the future - unpaid bills, catastrophic hypotheticals, etc. Such a mindset accelerates cortisol (stress hormone) which wears down the body. In short, idleness for too long empties your tank of all its fuel.

Proverbs 19:5 sheds light on a counterintuitive phenomenon regarding laziness. We presume that sleepiness makes people lazy. Yet, Solomon tells us that laziness makes people sleepy. Hang around all day for days upon days, and you'll find yourself more exhausted than the person working 50 hours weekly. Take machinery as an example. Usage of a machine keeps it functioning. No usage of a machine causes corrosion. A soul-probing question to answer today - Are you resting or are you rusting?

# SURVIVING FEELINGS WORKSHEET

## 1. Name it (Identification)

_____

_____

_____

_____

_____

_____

_____

_____

_____

## 2. Frame it (Validation)

_____

_____

_____

_____

_____

_____

_____

_____

_____

## 3. Tame it (Regulation)

_____

_____

_____

_____

_____

_____

_____

_____

_____

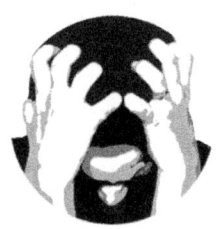

# I FEEL DISTRESSED

*We are troubled on every side, yet not distressed; we are perplexed, but not in despair;*

*Persecuted, but not forsaken; cast down, but not destroyed.*

II Corinthians 4:8-9

In December 1919, my papa Michele A. Caparrelli set foot in New York City with less than $20 and a few oven-roasted, fist-gripped chestnuts to warm his body from the 60-day oceanic voyage. When I probed my papa on why he left Italy, he replied, "Mussolini no good". Earlier that same year, Benito Mussolini arose as Duce of the Fascist party. My papa (a true progressive who despised fascism) read the handwriting on the wall much swifter than his neighbors and left without delay. Papa prophetically knew a hurricane was on the horizons; a wind of wrath that wouldn't surface until years later over Europe. What do bamboos do when the wind blows? They bend but don't break; that's my resilient papa.

Resilience is comprised of two characteristics - acceptance and adaptability. The first is acceptance. Papa accepted the reality that Italy would welcome an evil dictator, and there was no altering that fact. Acceptance squares off face to face with immutable realities - such as other people's choices - without pretending otherwise. Denial, the nemesis of acceptance, is what keeps people stuck and eventually ensues mental breakdowns. The second is adaptability. Papa took authority over what he could change while relinquishing what he couldn't. "I can't change Italy, but I can change me", he must have reasoned as he prepped his luggage. Adaptability means the readiness to embrace a new set of circumstances with a positive attitude. The species in the animal kingdom that survive the longest are not the strongest but the most adaptable.

Let's talk about II Corinthians 4. If you inquired the Apostle Paul about how he was feeling, he wouldn't have uttered flippantly, "Great!". There was no denial in Paul. Instead, he would have said, "Troubled, perplexed, persecuted...". Yet, if you asked Paul how he was functioning, he would have said, "I'm not destroyed. I'm moving forward!" Resilient people may feel bad but they function well. Their feelings don't overtake their functions. Like the Bamboo, they bend but they don't break.

# SURVIVING FEELINGS WORKSHEET

## 1. Name it (Identification)

_____
_____
_____
_____
_____
_____
_____
_____
_____
_____

## 2. Frame it (Validation)

_____
_____
_____
_____
_____
_____
_____
_____
_____
_____

## 3. Tame it (Regulation)

_____
_____
_____
_____
_____
_____
_____
_____
_____
_____

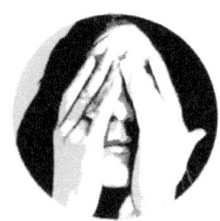

# I FEEL SEXUALLY IMPURE

*If our hearts condemn us, we know God is greater than our hearts,*

*and He knows everything.*

I John 3:20.

Survivors of sexual abuse often experience shame post-assault because of how their bodies responded during the act. In a study entitled, "Problems With Sexuality After Sexual Assault", the data revealed that 21% of women reported physical stimulation during the assault, 5% described an orgasm and 10% admitted sexual attraction to the perpetrator (Experts agree that the actual stats are much higher but shame is an inhibitor). Survivors often confuse biological sensations as an accurate reflection of their desires. "I must have wanted it" or "I feel like a slut" are just some of the shameful lies that survivors sadly believe.

If you've ever laughed while being involuntarily tickled, you know that the cackle was not a real depiction of your desires. The facts are, you hate being tickled. Laughing was merely a biological reaction to a bombardment of sensation to your nerve-endings. Similarly, any sexual stimulation you experienced during your assault was not what your soul wanted just as a person's laugh doesn't mean they enjoy being tickled. "Desire" happens within one region of our brain whereas "Arousal" occurs in a different part of our brain. Arousal alone is not a true portrayal of desire any more than crying equates to sadness when cutting an onion. What the soul desires and how the body feels are not always on the same page.

Within our passage of study, God is described as greater than our hearts for one simple reason - "He knows everything". Our hearts are deceived, hence an unqualified judge of our character. In some cases, our hearts mistake our biological reactions as an indication of our soul's yearnings. Oh, foolish heart! If you feel judged by your own heart, please know that there is One who is more eligible to assess you - Jesus Christ. Listen to what He proclaims rather than what your heart professes about you. In His eyes, under His blood, you are pure, chaste, and lovely.

---

Problems With Sexuality After Sexual Assault (National Library of Medicine, Van Berlo, 2000)

# SURVIVING FEELINGS WORKSHEET

## 1. Name it (Identification)

_____

_____

_____

_____

_____

_____

_____

_____

_____

## 2. Frame it (Validation)

_____

_____

_____

_____

_____

_____

_____

_____

_____

## 3. Tame it (Regulation)

_____

_____

_____

_____

_____

_____

_____

_____

_____

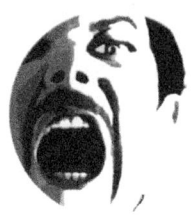

# I FEEL HATEFUL TOWARDS THE PEOPLE I HURT

*Amnon hated the sister he raped with intense hatred...Amnon said to her,*

*"Get up and get out!"*
II Samuel 13:15

Ashamedly, I confess to bullying a kid named Evan in elementary school. He towered over me but I leveraged my likable rep, wily mind, and silver tongue against him. Soon, a militia of kids rallied behind my antics (Years later, after initially hearing the gospel in a juvenile detention center, I repented from that mean streak). Equally despicable to the fact that I harassed him was the hatred that succeeded every verbal injury. I hated him for merely existing. Here's the kick in the head - The more I hurt him, the more I hated him.

In II Samuel 13:15, Amnon's treatment of his sister after he rapes her is not dissimilar to the innumerable cases of sexual violence that happen on the regular. "Get out of my face! I better never see you again, you piece of trash", is the typical disdainful follow-up. Are you sure that you hate that person at church, work, or within your family because they hurt you? Or, could you be hating them because you hurt them? Selah.

The University of Tokyo conducted a tell-tale experiment that involved the first group of participants (the shockers) administering electricity to the second batch of participants (the shocked). Researchers discovered that the more the shockers issued the shocks, the more they ranked the shocked participants as overreacting. Researchers theorized after further investigation that the "shockers" negatively altered their attitudes towards the "shocked" as over-reactive to eliminate cognitive dissonance (a fancy word for guilt). This theory sheds some light on why we hate the ones we hurt. It's easier for us to believe that the person we hurt is over-reactive or even bad, therefore deserved what they received than to face our savagery. Evan, please forgive me for hurting and hating you. God, forgive us for making the people we hurt "terrible" to excuse our actions against them as "tolerable".

---

Cognitive Dissonance Theory (American Psychological Association, Sakai, 1980)

# SURVIVING FEELINGS WORKSHEET

## 1. Name it (Identification)

_____
_____
_____
_____
_____
_____
_____
_____
_____
_____

## 2. Frame it (Validation)

_____
_____
_____
_____
_____
_____
_____
_____
_____
_____

## 3. Tame it (Regulation)

_____
_____
_____
_____
_____
_____
_____
_____
_____

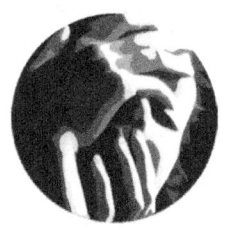

# I FEEL CONFUSED

*"Trust in the Lord with all your heart and lean not on your own understanding"*
Proverbs 3:5

A question you'll ask yourself throughout life - "How Will I Know?" How will I know that I'm in love? How will I know that I can trust this person? It's the question of epistemology. If you bank on your understanding to answer this, you'll end up in some serious quagmires. We just don't know what's good for us. Studies show infants prefer fatty, sweet foods over healthy foods. Babies only acquire a taste for healthy food from good parenting. Since Adam's fall from paradise, we don't know what's good for us.

Cross-modal perception (CMP) is a theory of psychology that shows how one sense easily influences another sense. For instance, people believe that food tastes better when they dine within a nice ambiance. The sight of a nice restaurant influences our taste buds. CMP reveals that our five senses interact, and even mislead one another. I once had my psych students survey other students on campus about how "kind" they believed a person was based on looking at a photo of their face. My students were instructed to hand people a hot cup of coffee when answering the question. Subjects who held the warm coffee believed the person in the photo was "kind" whereas those who held no coffee had no opinion. The warm sensation of the coffee influenced their judgment without the naive subjects even realizing it!

In Proverbs 3, the term "lean" means to "rest yourself upon something" like a man leaning into a cane. By forbidding us from leaning on our understanding, this verse implies that our perception is like a broken cane. Have you ever leaned into a broken cane? The inevitable outcome is falling flat on your face. That's the reality for those who rely upon their five senses to guide their decisions. Trusting in God is the only solid staff that upholds us in all matters. The hymnist said it right, "On Christ the solid rock I stand, all other ground is sinking sand".

# SURVIVING FEELINGS WORKSHEET

## 1. Name it (Identification)

_____

_____

_____

_____

_____

_____

_____

_____

_____

_____

## 2. Frame it (Validation)

_____

_____

_____

_____

_____

_____

_____

_____

_____

## 3. Tame it (Regulation)

_____

_____

_____

_____

_____

_____

_____

_____

_____

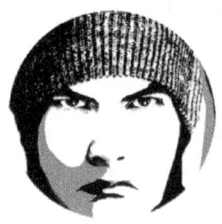

# I FEEL UNHAPPY WITH MY SPOUSE

*"Envy rots the bones"*

Proverbs 14:30

You have good reason to be unhappy! If your husband would pay more attention to you, you'd be just peachy. If you could move out of this dilapidated shanty, you'd be just dandy. A gazillion good reasons justify your miserable existence. But is your derelict hubby the bona fide reason why you're dissatisfied with life? As Mark Twain once stated, "Two reasons behind everything - the good reason we tell ourselves... and the real reason."

Consider this overlooked cause for unhappiness. Behavioral scientists performed an experiment involving two capuchins eating cucumbers (Brosnin&Dewall, 2003). For a while, the monkeys enjoyed their cucumbers. Then, the behavioral scientists introduced a second variable that changed everything. They gave the first monkey a handful of delicious grapes while handing the second monkey more cucumbers. After noticing monkey #1's grapes, monkey #2 chucked the cucumbers at the researcher's head! Suddenly, monkey #2 became bitterly dissatisfied with his portion. Social comparisons are at the root of many people's unhappiness. Facebook doesn't help since we're bombarded w/ images of other people's spouses & houses. Are you truly dissatisfied with what you have..or unhappy over what you don't have?

King Solomon handpicks an interesting metaphor to describe the effects of envy in Proverbs 14:30 - "the rotting of bones". Think about what happens when you fracture a bone. If you've ever broken your hip, every chair feels uncomfortable. If you've ever fractured your ankle, every shoe feels too tight. You'd be a fool to blame the chair or shoe for your unhappiness. That's how envy works - it corrodes what's beneath the surface so that you become uncomfortable with what's above the surface. Make no mistake about it- happiness or its counterpart unhappiness is an inside job.

---

Monkeys Reject Unequal Pay (Nature, Brosnan&Dewall, 2003)

# SURVIVING FEELINGS WORKSHEET

### 1. Name it (Identification)

_____

_____

_____

_____

_____

_____

_____

_____

_____

_____

### 2. Frame it (Validation)

_____

_____

_____

_____

_____

_____

_____

_____

_____

### 3. Tame it (Regulation)

_____

_____

_____

_____

_____

_____

_____

_____

_____

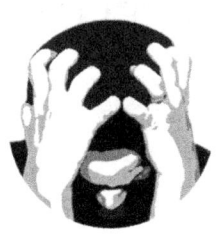

# I FEEL LIKE RELAPSING

*"After you have suffered a little while, the God of all grace will Himself*
*restore, confirm, strengthen and establish you"*
I Peter 5:10

I once embarked upon a road trip that required me to pass through a wretched city full of deplorable sights to arrive at a scenic location. My GPS made it clear that there was no easy way to my desirable destination without traversing through Sodom and Gomorrah. Likewise, the road to recovery from substance abuse entails hellish sights and sounds that cause many folks to give up before entering the promised land.

God designed your brain to produce a host of neurotransmitters for your emotional well-being. Neurotransmitters are your friends. Just to name a few, dopamine makes you feel pleasurable, GABA makes you peaceful and adrenaline makes you powerful. Now, let's talk about substance abuse. Substances mimic neurotransmitters at an exponential level - hence why you like drugs! Stimulants like cocaine impersonate Dopamine whereas sedatives like alcohol imitate GABA. Over time, your brain stops producing neurotransmitters on its own because it becomes dependent upon the substance for its production. The worse consequences of addiction are felt when you're not high or not drunk. You can no longer handle life on life's terms without feeling highly stressed or deeply depressed because of a lack of neurotransmitters.

When a person finally puts down the powder, the needle, or the bottle, the brain has lost its way. The suffering you experience in the initial stages of recovery is biological (in addition to being spiritual) - a depletion of neurotransmitters. Fortunately, after some time, the brain relearns how to produce these neurotransmitters on its own. Just as the scriptures promise, "After you suffer for a little while", strength returns. Emotional well-being is restored. Just like that voyage through the wretched city to enter the beautiful country, there is no promised land without passing through the valley of the shadow of death. If you feel like you're falling apart, just hang on for a little while because your chemicals will fall back into place.

# SURVIVING FEELINGS WORKSHEET

1. Name it (Identification)

_____
_____
_____
_____
_____
_____
_____
_____
_____

2. Frame it (Validation)

_____
_____
_____
_____
_____
_____
_____
_____
_____

3. Tame it (Regulation)

_____
_____
_____
_____
_____
_____
_____
_____
_____

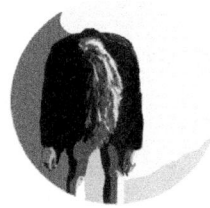

# I FEEL BAD ABOUT HOW I TREATED SOMEONE

*Therefore, if you are offering your gift at the altar and there remember that your brother or sister
has something against you, leave your gift there in front of the altar. First, go
and be reconciled to them; then come and offer your gift.*

Matthew 5:23-24

Gifted people get away with more infractions. Studies show that beautiful women are pardoned more readily for rule-breaking in the workplace. Funny people get away with more shenanigans on sports teams. Smart people get away with more unethical business practices in commerce. My mother received a letter from the school department when I was in elementary school requesting that I skip a grade due to results from a recent test; that same year, the teacher winked at me while I pulled all sorts of antics in class. Gifts such as beauty, intelligence, humor, and musicality are often used to camouflage a host of character defects.

A reason why gifted people get away with more infractions is a proven psychological phenomenon known as the halo effect. The halo effect is when we become so bedazzled, or star-struck, by someone's gifts that we overlook their character defects. It's called the halo ☐ effect because we whittle angels out of the people we admire. If you don't believe it's real, just talk with Jerry Sandusky's victims who had a tough time getting people to believe their stories. "Never could smart, athletic and charismatic Jerry be a pedophile", most faculty at Penn State reasoned. Giftedness whitewashes twistedness better than any Clorox bleach.

Within our passage of study, we encounter a gifted man. Now, his gift may take him places in society but it doesn't get him far with God. While offering his gift, it becomes apparent that he has hurt some people along the way. He remembers that certain folks have "ought" against him. God's imperative to the man shows us that He isn't interested in the gift of the giver; he's more concerned about the giver of the gift. Man looks at the outward appearance but the Lord sees the heart. Take heed, gifted people - if you prophesy like Jeremiah, exercise faith like Elijah, or preach like Spurgeon, but have not to love, you are nothing more than a clanging cymbal.

# SURVIVING FEELINGS WORKSHEET

## 1. Name it (Identification)

_____
_____
_____
_____
_____
_____
_____
_____
_____
_____

## 2. Frame it (Validation)

_____
_____
_____
_____
_____
_____
_____
_____
_____

## 3. Tame it (Regulation)

_____
_____
_____
_____
_____
_____
_____
_____
_____

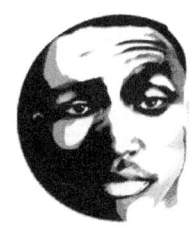

# I FEEL DISTANT FROM GOD

*And we all, who with unveiled faces contemplate the Lord's glory, are being transformed into his image with ever-increasing glory.*

II Corinthians 3:18

On November 22, 1963, an audience gathered in a small London playhouse to watch a comedic play written by David Lodge. During the play, a character tuned into the radio as part of the plot. To everyone's astonishment, a breaking announcement emitted through the radio that the United States president had been shot in Dallas, Texas. At that moment, true reality penetrated stage reality. Likewise, a spiritual experience is when divine reality breaks through temporal reality with astonishing announcements. Saints have such experiences during worship, listening to a sermon, or any practice of the presence of God.

A myriad of studies were performed over the last few decades to quantify the outcomes of a spiritual experience. One particular study using SPECT brain scans revealed that spiritual experiences (what we might call, "revelation") heightened activity in the frontal lobe. The frontal lobe is part of the brain whereby we envision, strategize and execute the highest forms of reasoning ( & colleagues, 2000). Other studies show a high release of growth hormones during a spiritual experience (Werner & colleagues, 1986). Growth hormones promote cell repairing and reproduction along with keeping your organs strong. When divine reality breaks through temporal reality, Zoe (spiritual life) enhances bios (biological life).

In II Corinthians 3, the worship experience is more than humdrum songs; instead, it ensures a personal transformation of the worshipper into the likeness of his/her object of adoration. Becoming like our God is the promise of every bona fide spiritual experience. When God came to us for the 1st time, He looked like us. When He returns the 2nd time, He expects us to look like Him. During worship, breaking news emits from heaven's tower about who He truly is and who we are becoming.

Meditation Not Only Reduces Stress But Here's How It Changes Your Brain (Harvard News, Schulte, 2015)

# SURVIVING FEELINGS WORKSHEET

## 1. Name it (Identification)

_____
_____
_____
_____
_____
_____
_____
_____
_____
_____

## 2. Frame it (Validation)

_____
_____
_____
_____
_____
_____
_____
_____
_____

## 3. Tame it (Regulation)

_____
_____
_____
_____
_____
_____
_____
_____
_____

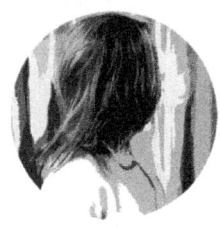

# I FEEL OPPOSED BY OTHERS

*The Pharisees were looking for a reason to accuse Jesus, so they watched him closely to see if he would heal him on the Sabbath. Jesus said to the man with the shriveled hand, "Stand up in front of everyone."...And Jesus healed the man.* Mark 3:1-6

Einstein's biggest critic was Phillip Lenard. Was he an anti-scientist? Nope. He was a physicist just like Al. Was he steeped in a different theory? Nope. He also invested his life in the atom. An all too common narrative in history - haters typically don't surface from the outside but usually arise from a kindred profession. Musicians often despise other musicians, hairdressers criticize other hairdressers, ministers compete with other ministers (of course, under the guise of "correct doctrine"), etc. Throw a party and invite two PhDs. They'll probably hit off with the plumber, but give each other skeptical glares throughout the evening. An underlying competition exists over who will be the champion of a particular territory. Pride says there's only room for one doctor in the house.

Behavioral Science research shows that you are more likely to bump heads with a person similar to you than different especially if you're aiming for the same goal. For instance, data analysis of the National Collegiate Athletic Association basketball teams found that a greater similarity among teams—in terms of geographic proximity, performance histories, and academic status—led to more intense experiences of rivalry (Kilduff et al., 2010). All this to resound the point, your greatest haters are usually wearing the same jersey as you.

Within our passage of study, Jesus is criticized, not by his constituents, but by his contemporaries. What did He do to warrant such an attack? He healed the sick, he fed the hungry, and he raised the dead. In short, he functioned at a level that his contemporaries couldn't operate on. Good ol' fashion jealousy, eh? Jesus pays the critics hardly any mind but focuses instead on his constituents. For those with lots of haters, ignore your critics and focus on the constituents. In the words of Stevie Wonder, "Preacher, keep on preaching. Teacher, keep on teaching. Until you reach the higher ground."

---

The Psychology of Rivalry (University of California, Kilduff, 2010)

# SURVIVING FEELINGS WORKSHEET

## 1. Name it (Identification)

_____
_____
_____
_____
_____
_____
_____
_____
_____
_____

## 2. Frame it (Validation)

_____
_____
_____
_____
_____
_____
_____
_____
_____

## 3. Tame it (Regulation)

_____
_____
_____
_____
_____
_____
_____
_____
_____

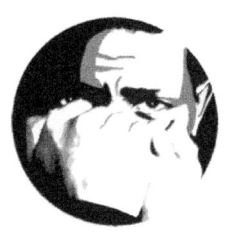

# I FEEL SCARED

*For God hath not given us the spirit of fear, but of power, and love, and a sound mind.*

II Timothy 1:7

Good advisors are level-headed. Bad advisors catastrophize. Catastrophizing means magnifying a manageable problem into a "no-way-out" nightmare. You'd be a fool to seek advice from catastrophizers. The outcome is high blood pressure and an awful migraine. Equally idiotic is the individual who gives too much credence to their fears. Fear is the worst advisor. Mulling over your fears is like looking through a magnifying glass at a small insect; fear renders a harmless spider into a ferocious dragon.

Fear disables our prefrontal cortex, the part of our brain that makes sensible decisions. Shmuel Lissek, PhD (2018) confirms this premise. Dr. Lissek devised a computer game where participants choose a short or long route to get from point A to point B. After playing for a while, the participants learned that the long route was the least sensible and usually ended in their destruction. When Lissek occasionally administered an electric shock (just a zap) to participants who chose the short route, participants selected the least sensible route to avoid the potential shock. Mind you, they ran the high risk of losing the game. Fear makes dummies out of otherwise geniuses.

II Timothy 1:7 contrasts the spirit of fear with a "sound mind". The Greek term for a sound mind is "sophronizo" which means a "sober mind, devoid of intoxication". The juxtaposition of this verse suggests that fear is like being inebriated, under the influence of a substance that impairs your judgment. Is fear telling you to run right now? Perhaps fear is telling you to withdraw your sword from its sheath? When General Patton was probed on how he executed such good judgment during World War II, he replied matter of factly, "I never took counsel from my fears".

---

Psychology of Fear (University of Minnesota, Lissek, 2019)

# SURVIVING FEELINGS WORKSHEET

## 1. Name it (Identification)

_____
_____
_____
_____
_____
_____
_____
_____
_____
_____

## 2. Frame it (Validation)

_____
_____
_____
_____
_____
_____
_____
_____
_____
_____

## 3. Tame it (Regulation)

_____
_____
_____
_____
_____
_____
_____
_____
_____

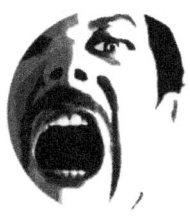

# I FEEL UNFORGIVING

*"Do not bear a grudge against anyone among your people,
but love your neighbor as yourself. I am the Lord."*
Leviticus 19:18

Taking on a task above your aptitude almost always results in stress. "I'll run the show today", you presumptuously tell the owner of the shop after the manager pulls a no-show. What were you thinking! Turmoil awaits you, the rookie, who presumes roles that surpass your skill-set. Did you know that holding a grudge is equivalent to presuming a role above your aptitude? For this reason, grudge-bearers are like high-strung rookies playing supervisors of the shop. Let me make this clearer for you...

Grudge-bearers are robe-wearers. Playing executioner won't even suffice for grudge-bearers - 'I gotta be the Judge!' Have you noticed (in books or movies) that when a man afflicts vengeance on a despised foe, he almost always makes his enemy look at him before he kills him! It's as if he's wanting the object of his fury to know, "I am the Judge! I am the Lord. Who's your daddy now?" Even in your own fantasies, how many times have you thought "I'll teach them a lesson". It's as if you want them to know the act of vengeance came from you. When you unmask a grudge, you'll find a yearning to play God. Neuroscience studies show a positive correlation between holding grudges, skyrocketing blood pressure and high cortisol levels (stress hormone). Why? Because presuming the highest office in the land always takes its toll on your health.

Regarding Leviticus 19:18, what strikes me is the last statement after God warns His people not to hold grudges - "I am the Lord" Such a proclamation not only reveals who God is but it exposes who grudge-bearers are trying to be. To borrow an Old Western phrase, God is saying to grudge-bearers, "There's only room for one sheriff in this town...and you ain't it".  If you want peace today, let go of the gavel, take off the robe, step down from the bench and let the true judge handle the matter. He's God all by Himself.

# SURVIVING FEELINGS WORKSHEET

1. Name it (Identification)

_____

_____

_____

_____

_____

_____

_____

_____

_____

_____

2. Frame it (Validation)

_____

_____

_____

_____

_____

_____

_____

_____

_____

_____

3. Tame it (Regulation)

_____

_____

_____

_____

_____

_____

_____

_____

_____

_____

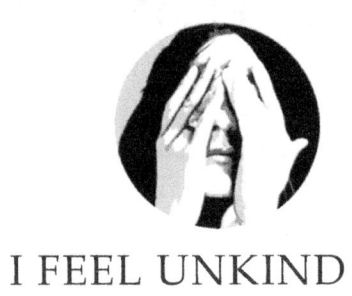

# I FEEL UNKIND

*Be kind to one another.*

Ephesians 4:32

Drowning people typically don't scream for their lives or gesticulate with their arms like in the movies. An individual drowns so quietly that it often goes unnoticed at a public beach crammed with swimmers. Likewise, the suicide of a relative or friend comes as a shock because the signs were so subtle. Such a person's agony was carefully concealed behind a cordial smile and a mild-mannered demeanor. As Thoreau stated, "The masses of men live lives of quiet desperation".

Suicidal ideation, from a neurological standpoint, is the activation of the "flight instinct" within the Amygdala of those who feel trapped. Van Heerigan and Marusic (2003) demonstrated that suicidal people "want out" as the prefrontal cortex disengages (the brain's problem-solving region) and the Amygdala fires off danger signals. Suicide derives from the inherently normal "flight instinct" - the same mechanism that influences people to leave unhappy jobs, marriages, etc. These dark feelings are equally biological as they are diabolical. Therefore, suicidal ideation can happen to anyone without forewarning. We all know what it feels like to "want out".

In Ephesians 4:32, the Apostle Paul exhorts us to practice indiscriminate kindness. Paul doesn't say, "Be kind to those who are hurting". He simply says "Be kind to one another". Since life takes its toll on everyone, kindness should be extended to anyone anywhere anytime. Albeit there's no simple solution for suicide prevention, kindness is the most feasible and perhaps powerful antidote. The most fatal myth we can believe is that the suicidal will carry out their plan no matter what we do. Kindness could inspire the person who thinks "I want out" to say "I'll remain in".

Understanding the Suicidal Brain (British Journal of Psychiatry, Van Heerigan&Marusic, 2003)

# SURVIVING FEELINGS WORKSHEET

## 1. Name it (Identification)

_____
_____
_____
_____
_____
_____
_____
_____
_____
_____

## 2. Frame it (Validation)

_____
_____
_____
_____
_____
_____
_____
_____
_____
_____

## 3. Tame it (Regulation)

_____
_____
_____
_____
_____
_____
_____
_____
_____
_____

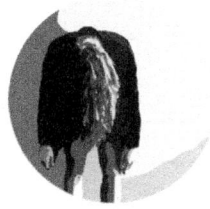

# I FEEL FORSAKEN

*A man of many companions may come to ruin, but there is One who stays closer than a brother.*

Proverbs 18:24

Survivors of childhood abuse feel hurt, not merely by their perpetrators, but by caretakers who turned a deaf ear to their cries. "How could so many have forsaken me? I have nightmares, not of my abuser, but hollow expressions from my parents, older siblings, teachers, and social workers who stare off into space while I bleed profusely", says one lady. Being utterly forsaken is mankind's greatest fear (hence the reason for Jesus' pinpointed promise, "I'll never forsake you"). Survivors live with the terror of being fundamentally alone throughout adulthood from the affect-residuals of a neglected childhood.

The Bystander Effect sheds some light (not all light) on why so many family and friends were heedless to your hurts. A dozen of social experiments since the 1960s were performed to confirm the Bystander Effect, a theory that states your likelihood of receiving help at a time of need decreases with more people present. A reason for this counterintuitive phenomenon is because bystanders gage the seriousness of your situation by how other bystanders respond. For instance, an older sibling might reason, "If mom doesn't think it's a big deal that my sister is always sad, then it must not be a big deal" or "My sister sees a counselor. Surely, the counselor would intervene if my sister was in trouble".

Long before behavioral science, King Solomon understood the "Bystander Effect". In Proverbs 18:24, Solomon accentuates the failure of the "many" to rescue you from your ruin while highlighting the faithfulness of the "One". The verse makes it clear that your rescuer will not arise from your beloved tribe. Even idyllic families are too handicapped by their own humanity to be your heroes. Being surrounded by hundreds of loving people offers no guarantee of safety for anyone, anywhere. Instead, Solomon points our attention to the "One"; a prophetic portrait of Jesus who may not stop every bad thing from happening but pledges to stick with you through it. All this to say, forgive family and friends for being handicapped by their own humanity, and stay close to the "One" who stays close to you.

# SURVIVING FEELINGS WORKSHEET

## 1. Name it (Identification)

_____
_____
_____
_____
_____
_____
_____
_____
_____
_____

## 2. Frame it (Validation)

_____
_____
_____
_____
_____
_____
_____
_____
_____
_____

## 3. Tame it (Regulation)

_____
_____
_____
_____
_____
_____
_____
_____
_____
_____

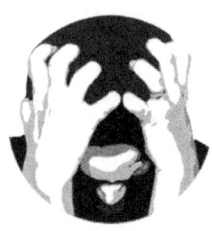

# I FEEL TEMPTED

*For you (your flesh) is dead, and you are hidden in Christ.*
Colossians 3:3

If you fell out of bed Friday night while sleeping, you're probably wondering how it happened. If you fell off the bed again last night, you're perplexed now. What's the deal with this chronic falling? Here's a novel thought - Maybe you fell off the bed because you slept too close to the edge. Let's apply this principle to temptations - pornography, substances, toxic romantic entanglements, etc. Frequent topples into such ditches indicate that you're walking too close to the edge.

Studies reveal that keeping your kryptonite at arm's length heightens your likelihood of sobriety. For instance, Cole, Dominick, and Balcetis (2021) conducted a simple experiment to prove this premise. Donut-lovers were granted the prerogative to sit wherever they wanted at a conference table with donuts on one side. Donut-lovers who seated themselves the furthest from their kryptonite ranked temptations substantially lesser than enthusiasts who sat right next to the orbits of delicious grease. A fairly simple principle is not applied enough - if you don't want to lay your hands on it, don't put your eyes on it. Step off the edge, my friend.

In Colossians 3:3, the prologue of Paul's statement (being dead in our fleshly desires) relies upon its epilogue (being hidden in Christ). To be hidden in Christ consists of being so wrapped up in life in Him that it distances you from everything contrary to His nature. Simple word this morning - You don't want to fall again into a temptation? Tuck yourself deeper into Christ.

---

Out of Reach and Under Control (Personality and Social Psychology, Cole et al., 2021)

# SURVIVING FEELINGS WORKSHEET

## 1. Name it (Identification)

_____
_____
_____
_____
_____
_____
_____
_____
_____
_____

## 2. Frame it (Validation)

_____
_____
_____
_____
_____
_____
_____
_____
_____
_____

## 3. Tame it (Regulation)

_____
_____
_____
_____
_____
_____
_____
_____
_____
_____

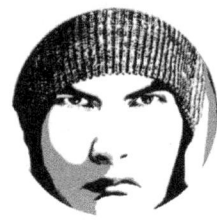

# I FEEL ANNOYED BY PEOPLE

*I make myself a slave (I accommodate myself) to all men that I might win some.*

I Corinthians 9:16

My wife Alicia and I are undoubtedly dissimilar. I'm intense; she's chill. I'm cerebral; she's super down to earth. I can be arrogant (the Almighty works overtime to keep me seemingly low); she's very humble without trying. Yet, the relationship works great like peas and carrots. Part of the reason why it works wonderfully is that variant spices often make up the best recipes - like a bag of salty popcorn with a blend of sweet Raisinets. The more paramount reason it works is that we find common ground everywhere. Conversely, the surest way of sabotaging what we have would be to focus on only the points of contention. Thank God we don't roll that way.

Are you butting heads with someone you love? Perhaps you're thinking, there's absolutely no common ground between my spouse and I, my sibling and I, my neighbor and I. Before you throw in the towel, consider this thought. The Human Genome Project was an international endeavor amongst scientists to study the DNA of countless people everywhere over 13 years. Over 3 billion genomes (genetic codes) were examined to capture a good picture of humans. The most astonishing finding of this project was that all humans are over 90 percent genetically similar! Those similarities are evident when you recognize our basic human needs/drives for love, belonging, respect, happiness, etc. Facts remain, you both at least chuckle watching Lucille Ball squish grapes with her feet and you both yearn to be loved, included, and respected.

Regarding I Corinthians 9, Paul is sagacious. He knows that relationships with people are not possible without establishing common ground. Hence, he embraces Jewish affinities when he's in company with the Jews. He probably references Abraham like he's an uncle from yesteryear when seated with a Pharisee. He nosedives into a dialogue about Caesar, government structures, and Italian marble when chilling with the Romans (Acts 22). All for one reason - to draw people closer to Christ. All of our relationships have the potential of manifesting God's glory when we step off the shaky ground and move onto common ground.

# SURVIVING FEELINGS WORKSHEET

## 1. Name it (Identification)

_____

_____

_____

_____

_____

_____

_____

_____

_____

_____

## 2. Frame it (Validation)

_____

_____

_____

_____

_____

_____

_____

_____

_____

_____

## 3. Tame it (Regulation)

_____

_____

_____

_____

_____

_____

_____

_____

_____

_____

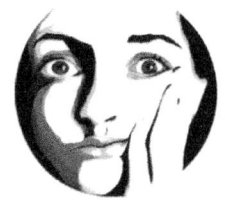

# I FEEL LIKE I PLAYED THE FOOL

*Above all else, Guard your heart...*

Proverbs 4:23

While seated alongside a mentor affectionately known as Uncle Arthur, a stranger walked in front of my car. "Michael, do you know that guy?", Uncle probed. "Nope", I replied. "Be careful with that stranger. He'll beat you for $20. But, be warier of your friends - they'll beat you for $20,000.". Uncle Arthur's warning, albeit cynical, wasn't a far cry from what the prophet Micah uttered centuries earlier, "A man's enemies will arise from his household (Micah 7:6). In my youthfulness, I supposed that Jesus' command to 'love your friends' and 'love your enemies' referred to two different people groups. Life taught me that Jesus was referring to the same people, just on different days of the week. Today's friends are often tomorrow's enemies.

Trust dilutes your discernment through a release of neurological chemicals. Behavioral scientists demonstrated through experiments that once oxytocin fires off in the brain, a person will carelessly assume vulnerable positions in a relationship (Kurowka, 2021, The Oxytocin-trust Link Experiment). Oxytocin is the "bonding hormone", initially released at birth, that makes us feel close to someone. The discharge of oxytocin inspires you to rent your home to a friend whom you never checked their credit report, or hire your best friend's wife to be your baby's nanny without any BCI. Oxytocin seduces you into trusting people without testing people. How is oxytocin released? Long before neuroscience, cultures throughout history figured out that a firm handshake makes business deals happen fast. A simple touch activates oxytocin.

Masterful architects know the fragile areas of their designs. Such architects place beams in the weak areas of any edifice they draft. In Proverbs 4:23, God orders a "guard" over the most vulnerable area of our makeup - the heart. Now, don't get it twisted - the heart is fragile for good reason. It is no mistake on God's part that our hearts are soft. Neither is oxytocin some "oops" chemical that happened accidentally in heaven's factory. God made us with vulnerable hearts for worship and fellowship. Only a soft substance is capable of bonding. Hard hearts are as useless as dried-up glue. Nonetheless, learn an invaluable lesson from every betrayal - guard your heart against its own risk factors, and don't let trusting stop you from testing.

---

Oxytocin-Trust Link (Frontiers in Neuroscience, Kurowka, 2021)

# SURVIVING FEELINGS WORKSHEET

## 1. Name it (Identification)

_____

_____

_____

_____

_____

_____

_____

_____

_____

_____

## 2. Frame it (Validation)

_____

_____

_____

_____

_____

_____

_____

_____

_____

## 3. Tame it (Regulation)

_____

_____

_____

_____

_____

_____

_____

_____

_____

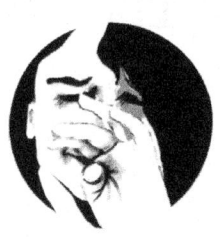

# I FEEL HOPELESS

*We glory in our sufferings because we know that suffering produces perseverance, perseverance produces character and character produces hope.*

Romans 5:3

Kintsugi is an ancient Japanese art that involves making the most of broken pottery. Practitioners of this unique art refuse to hide the flaws of a cracked vase; instead, they rejoin the broken pieces together with a lacquer mixed with powdered gold, silver, and platinum. The final product reflects the vase's exquisite beauty while still preserving its painful history. Multiple case studies in behavioral science indicate people who've extracted beauty out of their painful history. PTSD is not the only fate of those of you who've suffered immensely; PTG (Post-Traumatic Growth) awaits you. PTG is characterized by a greater appreciation for life and overall strength.

So, what are PTG folks doing to shovel their way out of PTSD? No simple answer exists for this question, but one common theme emerges from the research - lessening experiential avoidance. Kashan and Kane (2011) examined a sample of people who underwent either a sudden death of a loved one, a severe automotive accident, an episode of violence, and a natural disaster. Researchers discovered that the greater the distress, the more neurological evidence of PTG - but ONLY in those participants with low levels of experiential avoidance. Experiential avoidance means relying on a handful of defense mechanisms that enable you to block out the pain. Researchers discovered that folks who avoided the pain in the short term exacerbated their stress in the long term. PTG folks are like Kintsugi artists who refuse to camouflage their cracks; instead, they reflect an exquisite beauty amalgamated with their painful history.

In Romans 5:3, the Apostle Paul employs an eye-opening word to describe the overcomer's response to pressure - perseverance. The Greek term for perseverance, hypomonen, means to remain under something until its endpoint. It paints the picture of working through the pain of an ordeal until the moment of breakthrough. It's the utter opposite of defense mechanisms that enable us to avoid suffering. Romans 5:3 shows that when we persevere, we don't just go through trials; we grow through trials. Learn the art of Kintsugi.

---

Post-Traumatic Distress and the Presence of Post-Traumatic Growth
(Personality and individual differences, Kashdan and Kane, 2011)

# SURVIVING FEELINGS WORKSHEET

## 1. Name it (Identification)

_____
_____
_____
_____
_____
_____
_____
_____
_____

## 2. Frame it (Validation)

_____
_____
_____
_____
_____
_____
_____
_____
_____

## 3. Tame it (Regulation)

_____
_____
_____
_____
_____
_____
_____
_____
_____

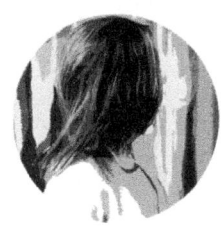

# I FEEL CLOSED OFF FROM PEOPLE

*Do not neglect to show hospitality to stranger.*
Hebrews 13:2

What sparks friendships? Some say it's chemistry; inexplicable energy that flows without rhyme or reason between two people. Others say it's mutuality; that moment the two of you realize you share a kindred personality, story, or preference. Others say it's adversity; a common plight that draws the oddest people together. Like Shakespeare said, "Misery makes strange bedfellows." But what if the sparks that ignite friendships are more random than reasonable? Consider the following legendary social experiment from the 1950s known as the Westgate Study that speaks volumes about what sparks friendships....

In 1950, social scientists examined communal apartment buildings known as Westgate to understand what sparks friendships. In short, social scientists asked the Westgate participants to list their closest friends, and discovered that 2/3rds of these pals lived in the same building! 41% lived in units adjacent to their unit whereas only 10% lived in units on other floors. These results paved the way for a litany of other experiments that established a psychological phenomenon known as the law of propinquity. The law of propinquity asserts that we are most likely to forge friendships with people closest in proximity. Sorry to burst your bubble, but friends are not always the people you adore the most but the folks who got there first!

Hospitality is what makes the Christmas story so remarkable. The term, hospitality, in Greek is PhiloXenos, an oxymoronic word that abrasively rubs against our human instincts. The prefix, Philos, means "loving someone like a brother." The suffix, Xenos, means "the perfect stranger". In summary, hospitality means to love the perfect stranger like a beloved brother. Isn't that precisely what happened through the incarnation of Jesus? He and I were perfect strangers from opposite ends of the spectrum; He is Holy whereas I am filthy. Yet, through the incarnation, He extends a friendly handshake. Be like your Savior by showing hospitality; spark relations with a perfect stranger from the other side of the track.

# SURVIVING FEELINGS WORKSHEET

1. Name it (Identification)

_____
_____
_____
_____
_____
_____
_____
_____
_____
_____

2. Frame it (Validation)

_____
_____
_____
_____
_____
_____
_____
_____
_____
_____

3. Tame it (Regulation)

_____
_____
_____
_____
_____
_____
_____
_____
_____
_____

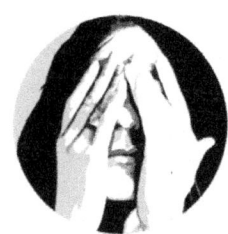

# I FEEL SENSITIVE

*Consider what God has done: Who can straighten what he has made crooked?*

Ecclesiastes 7:13

A sensor is the primary mechanism of a thermometer, a thin bulb that reads the hotness or coldness of a room. Such an apparatus is easily breakable, yet you wouldn't want it any other way. If it were hard like a hammer, it would never fulfill its function of discerning temperatures. Sensitivity is an integral part of its design, and the reason it can read a room so easily. Likewise, highly sensitive people (which comprise approx. 20% of the population) are often criticized as being too "thin-skinned" yet FMRIs reveal functionality behind such sensitivity. MRIs indicate accelerated activity in the insular and the inferior frontal gyrus, areas of the brain that make highly sensitive people more aware of interpersonal affairs and empathetic toward those in distress (Brain and Behavior, July 2014). Other studies show approx 50 distinctive genes involved in high sensitivity. Like the thermometer's sensor, sensitivity is not a character flaw but an integral part of the way some people were designed.

Putting the gift of sensitivity to use is partly what keeps it from morphing into a handicap. Let's face it – being overly sensitive can easily lend itself to rumination, depression, and anxiety. One moment, you discern your BFF is in distress. The next moment, you're ruminating over what you did to cause their agony. Sensitivity can take a sharp left fairly quickly. Conversely, utilizing sensitivity for what it's for could keep you from stepping into these psychological nooses. A growing body of research indicates that an act of kindness towards people in distress is a protective factor against anxiety and depression. Perhaps your intuition that Sal or Sally is hurting means a thoughtful card, an invitation to the spa, or a meal made with love.

King Solomon's opening phrase, "Consider what God has done", accredits the Almighty as the reason behind certain "crooked" parts of creation. Not everything "crooked" is the outcome of being damaged by mother nature or human nature; some "crooked" things were made that way by their Maker. Next time you criticize yourself as being defective, take heed to Solomon's words. Consider that this "crookedness" might be exactly how God made it to be? A sensor would lose all functionality if it lost its sensitivity.

The Highly Sensitive Brain (Acevado, Brain and Behavior, 2014)

# SURVIVING FEELINGS WORKSHEET

## 1. Name it (Identification)

_____
_____
_____
_____
_____
_____
_____
_____
_____
_____

## 2. Frame it (Validation)

_____
_____
_____
_____
_____
_____
_____
_____
_____
_____

## 3. Tame it (Regulation)

_____
_____
_____
_____
_____
_____
_____
_____
_____
_____

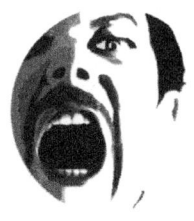

# I FEEL HEATED

*Be angry but sin not.*
Ephesians 4:26

1. Back up from the immediate company. Anger is the result of your amygdala - the survival mechanism in your brain - warning you of imminent danger. Whether an explosion erupts from within or without, anger works like a smoke alarm telling you it's time to get out of the building.

2. Breath. Deep breaths have been proven under FMRIs to decelerate the amygdala in times of heated passion. Solomon promises that if we "slow down our anger, we will gain much understanding" (Proverbs 14:29). Breathing slows it down. You'll find a couple of incidences in the gospels whereby "Jesus sighed", a deep breath at moments of high stress to slow down (Mark 8:12, 7:34).

3. Look beneath the surface. Anger is like the red flashing light on your dashboard that indicates something under the hood has gone wrong. Underneath the hood, you'll either find hurt, disappointment, sadness, fear, or some other more vulnerable emotion. Hence the reason God asks Cain "why are you so angry?" (Genesis 4:6).

4. Submit yourself to the Almighty. Satan is a pyromaniac who shows up at every fire to use the flames for his agenda - destruction. In moments of anger, sin is not far off. The Apostle James tells us that the posture of submission to God gives us leverage over the evil one (James 4:7).

5. Work towards justice. Anger, at its fundamental level, is a boost of adrenaline that energizes you for a task. Research conducted by the University of Michigan shows that anger makes people better negotiators, more creative in problem-solving, and more assertive overall. The key is, discerning what injustice sparked your anger and how to work towards resolving that injustice for all humanity.

# SURVIVING FEELINGS WORKSHEET

## 1. Name it (Identification)

_____

_____

_____

_____

_____

_____

_____

_____

_____

## 2. Frame it (Validation)

_____

_____

_____

_____

_____

_____

_____

_____

_____

## 3. Tame it (Regulation)

_____

_____

_____

_____

_____

_____

_____

_____

_____

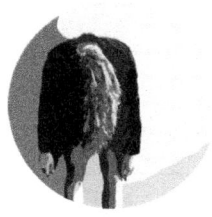

# I FEEL SHAMED

*They exclaimed, "Surely, He was the son of God."*
Matthew 27:64

We care what people think. Social media venues would flatline if this wasn't true. There would be zero selfies. In a recent survey conducted amongst 166 university students, 70% of respondents claimed they'd rather have their arms amputated than forever branded a "Nazi", and over 1/3rd would rather "die now" than be known as a pedophile (Vonasch, 2017). Why? Because we care what people think. Even the public statement, "I don't care what people think of me", is an inadvertent admission that you care what people think, or else you wouldn't care that others know that you don't care (Read that again). Like it or not, you are a social being that derives your identity from group status.

Fewer things are more distressing than watching your name dragged through the mud you never traversed. Catching wind of false accusations made against you, whether whispered by cowards or blasted by social media bullies, takes its toll on your wellbeing. Research shows a definite correlation between being shamed and suicide (Wiklander et al. 2012). It's no surprise that Jesus stated that slanderers will be convicted as murderers on the day of judgment since you snuff out a person's spirit by attacking their name. So, how do you clear your name when this happens? I've been there many times, so I speak from lots of experience.

Dubbed a liar yet He was the essence of truth. Depicted as a blasphemer yet He was God himself. Despite the onslaught, He advanced even as the Romans and Jews nailed him to an old rugged tree. A few seconds after He gave up the ghost, His haters shockingly professed, "Surely He was the Son of God". Do you want to clear your name? Onward and upward in your mission, and the hour shall come when slanderers will eat their words...but usually after you've shown class and courage under fire.

---

Death Before Dishonor (Social Psychological and Personality, Vonasch, 2017)

# SURVIVING FEELINGS WORKSHEET

1. Name it (Identification)

_____

_____

_____

_____

_____

_____

_____

_____

_____

_____

2. Frame it (Validation)

_____

_____

_____

_____

_____

_____

_____

_____

_____

_____

3. Tame it (Regulation)

_____

_____

_____

_____

_____

_____

_____

_____

_____

_____

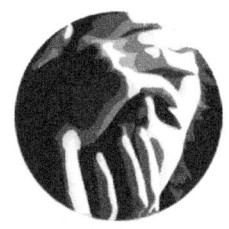

# I FEEL UNHEARD

*Only let your conversation be as the gospel of Christ:*
*that whether I come and see you, or else be absent, I may hear of your affairs.*

Philippians 1:27

A good dialogue with someone is like playing ping pong; a back and forth momentum that sharpens your senses. Good dialogues are reciprocal with a sweet balance of hearing and sharing. Following a good dialogue, I usually feel inspired. But some conversations lack reciprocity. Only one person talks incessantly about themselves without exhibiting any curiosity about the other party. These conversations don't leave you feeling inspired but tired. I don't even dub it a dialogue. I call it "a monologue in the presence of witnesses".

A recent study conducted at the University of Delaware indicated that conversations with a person who interrupts frequently or monopolizes the time result in negative views of that person afterward (Ann Manser, 2020). We, humans, possess inherent needs to understand and be understood, to know and be known. We engage in dialogue to have both needs fulfilled. One-way conversations (a.k.a., monologues in the presence of a witness) leave us feeling emotionally deprived. How much fun would it be to play ping-pong with someone who catches the ball, holds it for ten minutes, and rambles rather than hitting it back to you?

Perhaps what made the Apostle Paul so influential amongst his constituents was his desire to know them. If any historical character had something to contribute to a conversation, it'd be the Apostle Paul. A Roman citizen, a Pharisee amongst Pharisees and, most notably, an eyewitness of the resurrected Christ, Paul could tell you stories that would have you at the edge of your seat. With so much to share, Paul still exhibited a desire to hear. Interactions with Paul would leave any man desirous to know the Christ that lived within him. The adage stands true, people don't care what you know until they know that you care.

Don't Touch That Phone (University of Delaware, Masner, 2020)

# SURVIVING FEELINGS WORKSHEET

## 1. Name it (Identification)

_____
_____
_____
_____
_____
_____
_____
_____
_____

## 2. Frame it (Validation)

_____
_____
_____
_____
_____
_____
_____
_____
_____

## 3. Tame it (Regulation)

_____
_____
_____
_____
_____
_____
_____
_____
_____

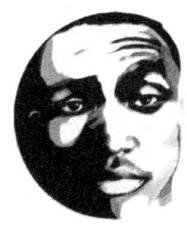

# I FEEL LIKE I WANT TO BE FREE

*It is for freedom that Christ has set you free. Stand firm, then,*

*and do not let yourself be burdened again by a yoke of slavery.*

Galatians 5:1

I've been attending 12 Step Meetings since the 1990s, and I can tell you that coffee and/or pastries become quite the obsession. I've witnessed many men triumph over alcoholism (thank God!) while morphing into jittery, caffeine-infused dudes with bellies draped over their waste buckles. "I haven't had a drink in five years but can't put down the Twinky", I'm waiting for someone to confess while slurping their extra-large Macchiato. To borrow a phrase from Ann Lamont, "Just because you've shaken a certain monkey off your back doesn't mean you've left the circus."

In a nationally representative study, behavioral scientists discovered that remission from a substance abuse disorder increased the onset likelihood of a new addiction (Blanco et al, 2014, Testing the drug substitution switching model). In other words, many folks don't kick addictions but merely switch addictions. In Galatians 5:1, Paul warns the people of God of leaving one form of captivity to merely enter another form of captivity. By the end of Galatians, Paul essentially tells the people what my pastor, Pasco Manzo, always told me "Let nothing master you but the Master (Jesus)".

Once upon a time, a young boy helped his pet frog kick an addiction to cookies by hiding the sugary treats on the top shelf where its legs weren't strong enough to leap. Nonetheless, the frog made every effort to reach those cookies. Every morning, he jumped higher and higher. Until one day, he realized he was never gonna reach those darn cookies. The frog finally gave up. The boy said to his frog, "Finally, you kicked your addiction to cookies! I'm so proud of you. What will you do now?". The frog replied, "I think I'll bake a cake"

Testing the Drug Substitution Switching Addictions (NCBI, Blanco, 2015)

# SURVIVING FEELINGS WORKSHEET

1. Name it (Identification)

_____

_____

_____

_____

_____

_____

_____

_____

_____

2. Frame it (Validation)

_____

_____

_____

_____

_____

_____

_____

_____

_____

3. Tame it (Regulation)

_____

_____

_____

_____

_____

_____

_____

_____

_____

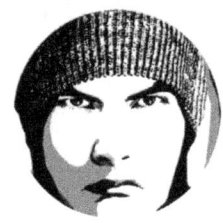

# I FEEL DISTANT FROM MY SPOUSE

*Come, let us take our fill of love until the morning. Let us delight ourselves with love.*
*My husband is not at home, for he has gone on a long journey.*
Proverbs 7:18-19

Marital affairs often exhibit the euphoria of love. A feedback loop occurs between dopamine, norepinephrine, and oxytocin that makes the cheater feel like their hearts have been hijacked by some love interest. Dopamine releases pleasure, norepinephrine arouses the five senses and oxytocin makes one feel close to someone. Merely the smell of Casanova's cologne, or a smirk from Delilah, triggers this triad of neurotransmitters into a loop that makes the subject loopy. Notice in Proverbs that the adulterous woman describes her affair, not as "lust" but "love". The fog gets so thick that the driver assumes they're heading into bliss when they're driving off a cliff (Stats show that most of these love affairs end badly).

Cheater's fog, a real neurological state of mind, blinds a person in two ways. First, the cheater falls prey to the Halo Effect whereby they perceive their love interest as an angel who can do no wrong. The cheater lazar focuses on the admirable traits of Casanova or Delilah while dismissing any apparent character defects. Second, the cheater falls prey to the Horn Effect whereby they perceive their current spouse as the devil. The cheater magnifies every mistake the spouse makes into an offense worthy of capital punishment, all to eliminate their guilt.

In one brief statement, Proverbs 7 sheds light on the people most susceptible to cheater's fog. The adulterous woman says, "my husband is away on a long journey". Interestingly enough, studies show that affairs are the highest amongst people with emotional and/or physical distance in their marriages (Russel et al., 2013, Attachment insecurity and infidelity). Make no mistake about it, the surest protection against cheater's fog is to love the one you're with. Do what must be done to bridge the gap between you and your spouse today with the help of God and the people of God.

# SURVIVING FEELINGS WORKSHEET

## 1. Name it (Identification)

_____
_____
_____
_____
_____
_____
_____
_____
_____

## 2. Frame it (Validation)

_____
_____
_____
_____
_____
_____
_____
_____
_____

## 3. Tame it (Regulation)

_____
_____
_____
_____
_____
_____
_____
_____
_____

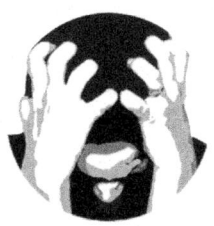

# I FEEL RUSHED

*Esau said to Jacob, "Quick, let me have some of that red stew! I'm famished!"*
Genesis 25:30

Rushing you into buying the product is the trick of the tempter (Satan) "This offer expires today", says the car salesman. Tempters hope for you to submit to that rush of euphoria flooding through your veins at the sight of something you like. In the rush of the moment, the feeling of "I got to have it or I'll die" prevails. But it's all the result of biology gone mad!

A proven strategy for overcoming temptation is to slow down, inhale and exhale. Brain mappings show the prefrontal cortex engaging when a person breathes. The prefrontal cortex is the center of executive reasoning where you weigh out the pros and cons of every decision. Remember the Analyst from the introduction of this book! Make it a habit that when the tempter presses the gas pedal, you apply the brakes. Allow your right mind to thoroughly assess a decision without the interference of that rush.

The first time I read this story about Jacob and Esau, I dismissed it as a fable no truer than Disney's fabrications. In my cynical mind, I reasoned, "Who would sell their birthright, something so valuable, for a bowl of stew?". But after reading enough headlines about pastors, celebrities, and athletes who nearly sabotaged their lives for a moment of pleasure, I realized that this story rings true. Every man is capable of selling their birthright for a bowl of stew, providing they feel rushed like Esau and it's the right flavor of soup.

# SURVIVING FEELINGS WORKSHEET

## 1. Name it (Identification)

_____
_____
_____
_____
_____
_____
_____
_____
_____
_____

## 2. Frame it (Validation)

_____
_____
_____
_____
_____
_____
_____
_____
_____

## 3. Tame it (Regulation)

_____
_____
_____
_____
_____
_____
_____
_____
_____

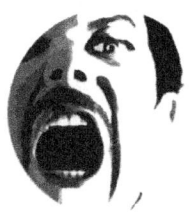

# I FEEL DEFENSIVE

*We have divine power to demolish strongholds. We demolish arguments and every pretension*
*that sets itself up against the knowledge of God.*
II Corinthians 10:4-5

I overheard a young man inquire of his pastor, "What sin is chief of all - pride, lust, greed?". The minister sagaciously replied, "The sin you're most defensive about". Defensiveness is a reflex that inhibits the heart from receiving truth. Sure, the truth sets you free eventually, but it ticks you off initially. Your soul's watchdog flaunts its fangs at the intruder of truth, wishing to scare it away. The most hazardous sin in your life is the one you bark the loudest about when confronted.

No wonder the scriptures describe every ungodly pattern of thought as a "stronghold". A stronghold is a defensive fort during battle, keeping its inhabitants safe. Consider the following strongholds, a.k.a. Defensive Mechanisms, that inhibit you from hearing the truth.

<u>PROJECTION</u> - You spot defects in others that, ironically, you possess. Your subconscious mind pulls the proverbial wool over your eyes, making you think what you notice belongs to your neighbor but it's your own plank; e.g. you think others are jealous of you, when in fact you're jealous of them. You spot it because you got it.

<u>DEFLECTION</u> - You're preoccupied with other people's habits, hang-ups, and hurts so that you have no time to look in the mirror at your own. .

<u>RATIONALIZATION</u> - You make wrongs right within your head through justifying and rationalizing. These rationales are deceptions that enable you to live more comfortably with your sin. Another way of pronouncing Rationalize is Rational-Lies.

May the kindness of God bypass our defenses and lead us into repentance.

# SURVIVING FEELINGS WORKSHEET

1. Name it (Identification)

_____
_____
_____
_____
_____
_____
_____
_____
_____
_____

2. Frame it (Validation)

_____
_____
_____
_____
_____
_____
_____
_____
_____
_____

3. Tame it (Regulation)

_____
_____
_____
_____
_____
_____
_____
_____
_____

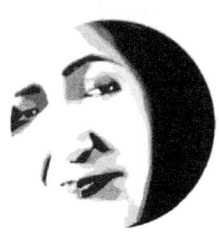

# I FEEL SUSPICIOUS

*The righteous choose their friends carefully.*

Proverbs 12:26

Three times in my life, I had a pit in my stomach about someone's trustworthiness, yet I went forth with forging a close relationship with that person anyway. In each case, my initial discernment proved right after I experienced major betrayal at the hands of the suspicious character. Why didn't I listen to my discernment? All three situations share one common denominator. The Judas in my stories possessed one or more characteristics familiar to me or bore some striking resemblance to my family of origin. May I submit to you that we are most easily bewitched by what's familiar to us?

An interesting study performed by St. Andrew's University revealed that we are fond of people who physically resemble our parents. The study showed that participants were less attracted to youthful faces when raised by parents who were older than 30 years old, and vice versa (2002). Other similar studies show that we are drawn to people who possess similar cultural attributes or personality traits to our beloved relatives. This causes us to fall prey to the "law of least effort". The law of least effort means that we seek short-cuts, or heuristics, in making decisions about people's character. Making a solid decision about someone's character requires too much time and effort so we rely upon heuristics - such as familiar attributes - to guide our decisions.

Wise Solomon cautions us to choose our friends "carefully" in Proverbs 12:26. The Hebrew term for "careful" alludes to spies that survey a particular land of interest. When spies survey the territory, they not only examine the land's fruitfulness but take into account any potential threats. By employing this Hebrew term for "careful", Solomon warns us to conduct a thorough assessment of someone's character before forging a close companionship. Are you falling prey to the law of least effort, or are you making careful decisions when choosing your companions? If you've prayed for protection, know that God typically answers that prayer by giving us discernment. Use it or suffer the perils from neglecting it.

---

Facial Attractiveness Judgments... (Proc Biological Science, Perrett, 2002)

# SURVIVING FEELINGS WORKSHEET

## 1. Name it (Identification)

_____
_____
_____
_____
_____
_____
_____
_____
_____
_____

## 2. Frame it (Validation)

_____
_____
_____
_____
_____
_____
_____
_____
_____
_____

## 3. Tame it (Regulation)

_____
_____
_____
_____
_____
_____
_____
_____
_____

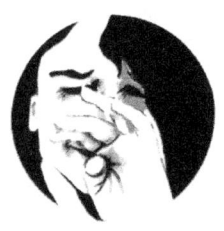

# I FEEL FED UP WITH CHURCH

*"You unbelieving generation," Jesus replied,*
*"How long shall I put up with you? Bring the boy to me."*
Matthew 17:17

Whenever the demand is too high for a particular circuit, a fuse blows and the power goes out. Here and there, the church exhibits itself powerless in moments when people are in dire need. Suicidal teens, destitute single parents, sexually confused young adults, grief-stricken widows and scores of shackled vagabonds storm into the sanctuary for help, only to find that the proverbial lights are out. Studies indicate that clergy is the most preferred first-responders to a crisis yet among helping professionals, the ones who feel the most ill-equipped. What a conundrum! May I submit to you that the church's fuses occasionally blow out because the demand exceeds the resources?

The number of Americans ages 18-29 who have no religious affiliation has nearly quadrupled over the last 3 decades, and 59% of millennials raised in a church vamoosed. Why? Folks are disappointed with the church for not coming through at critical moments. But, there are two pivotal factors easily forgotten, the second being a real game-changer. The first factor is that the church is comprised of finite beings; the term finite connotes limitations. Clergy and laypeople often lack the supply (time, energy, resources) to keep up with the demand. The second game-changing factor....well, read on.

In Matthew 17, a father escorts his tormented son to Jesus' disciples, a.k.a., the church, and encounters a band of poor physicians. What do you do when the church doesn't work? The father pursues the Savior himself. Jesus replies, "Bring the boy to me". Perhaps God is saying to you, "Never mind the brother or sister next to you. Bring your problem to me". If you've been disappointed by what's in the pews, then hit the altars. Thankfully, pews are not the only fixtures in the sanctuary. When the power goes out in my house, I don't tear out every socket. I simply go to the power box.

# SURVIVING FEELINGS WORKSHEET

## 1. Name it (Identification)

_____

_____

_____

_____

_____

_____

_____

_____

_____

_____

## 2. Frame it (Validation)

_____

_____

_____

_____

_____

_____

_____

_____

_____

## 3. Tame it (Regulation)

_____

_____

_____

_____

_____

_____

_____

_____

_____

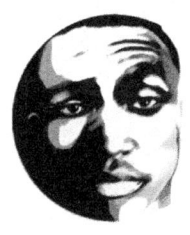

# I FEEL LIKE BLAMING SOMEONE

*The next day John saw Jesus coming toward him, and said,*
*"Behold, the Lamb of God, who takes away the sin of the world!"*
John 1:29

If a dude is justly fired from his job, yet refuses to acknowledge sloppy work ethic, dragging his boss' name through the mud is very likely. If a person's marriage ends from infidelity, yet that person denies messing around, bashing their ex is highly probable. Scapegoating is defined as shifting personal culpability and corresponding guilt to someone else. In the words of a song from yesteryear, "Blame it on the rain, blame it on the stars....Whatever you do, don't blame it on you".

Freud popularized the theory when noting that a patient was most critical of his neighbor at moments when he harbored guilt over his hang-ups. Another historic study from the 1800s revealed that Southern farmers treated slaves most harshly when their profits suffered from their negligence. Scapegoating theory suggests that people are often angry to the degree that they feel consciously or subconsciously guilty. Harbored guilt exhibits itself through a long, boney finger pointed at someone else.

John the Baptist beholds the Lamb of God rather than a human goat to expunge his sins. The prophet models the only way to propitiate our conscience of all guilt - accept by faith what Jesus did for you on Calvary. When awakened to the knowledge of your gross shortcomings, you have one or two choices - look to the cross, or put someone else on the cross. I assure you, the lamb is more effective than the goat.

# SURVIVING FEELINGS WORKSHEET

## 1. Name it (Identification)

_____

_____

_____

_____

_____

_____

_____

_____

_____

## 2. Frame it (Validation)

_____

_____

_____

_____

_____

_____

_____

_____

_____

## 3. Tame it (Regulation)

_____

_____

_____

_____

_____

_____

_____

_____

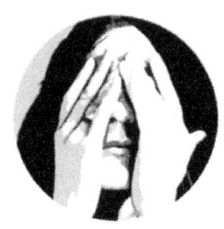

# I FEEL HINDERED

*But Jesus called them unto him, and said,*
*Suffer little children to come unto me, and forbid them.*
Matthew 19:14

Plants only blossom as big as their pots permit. Biologists discovered that plants bloom over 40% larger by simply setting them in a sizable jardiniere. Likewise, a child's initiative, intellect, and integrity bloom to the degree that their environments allow. Beethovens and Abe Lincolns are not solely outcomes of an exceptional disposition, but the offshoots of a fertile atmosphere. Take note that both champions were nurtured by some loving guardian. To a certain degree, men and women are what their mommies and daddies made of them when they were seedlings (of course, free will plays the most pivotal role).

An abusive environment is a puny pot that hinders a child's growth. I often wonder how many world-changers by disposition sputtered into drug addicts because of being reared in a vessel shattered along the seams. Neuroscience reveals that victims of early childhood abuse possess brain injuries equivalent to physical head traumas even when they've never hit their heads. Brain mappings indicate severe delays in the hippocampus (memory), cerebral vermis (emotional regulation), and the prefrontal cortex (logic) amongst victims of early childhood abuse. Today, if you meet a crack-pot, chances are they grew up in a cracked pot.

"Suffer the little children", Jesus' statement to the austere disciples, is an ancient way of saying, "Let the children go!" Let the kids play when they feel silly. Let the kids cry when they feel sad. Let the kids talk when something weighs heavy on their minds. No telling what shall become of your offspring when you forbid them not from growing. And to all the crack-pots abroad (my peeps!), suffer your inner-child. The time is never too tardy to let your child out to experience the magical kingdom of God.

# SURVIVING FEELINGS WORKSHEET

## 1. Name it (Identification)

_____
_____
_____
_____
_____
_____
_____
_____
_____
_____

## 2. Frame it (Validation)

_____
_____
_____
_____
_____
_____
_____
_____
_____
_____

## 3. Tame it (Regulation)

_____
_____
_____
_____
_____
_____
_____
_____
_____

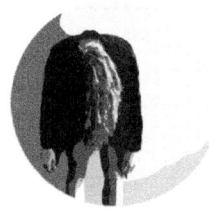

# I FEEL SELF-DOUBTFUL

*For she said within herself, "If I may but touch his garment, I shall be whole."*
Matthew 9:21

The most pivotal conversation you engage in - next to your chats with Jesus - is the talk you have with yourself. Survivors of childhood abuse often talk to themselves in the same tone as their abusers berating them. News alert - your perpetrators succeeded in massacring your soul when their words become your thoughts. Healing from the damage of sexual abuse includes changing the channel of your self-talk to a more pleasant, self-edifying tune. The dial is in your hands.

Self-talk bears significant effects on your life outcomes. Whether you tell yourself you can or can't accomplish a particular task, you're right! Studies in positive psychology indicate that the subtlest shifts in what we say to ourselves make a difference in our performance. Researchers suggest the following shifts (Mayo Clinic Staff, 2019) -

* Instead of "I've never done it before," try "It's an opportunity to learn something new."
* Instead of "It's too complicated," try "I'll tackle it from a different angle."
* Instead of "I'm not going to get any better at this," try "I'll give it another try."
* Instead of "I don't have the resources," try "Necessity is the mother of invention."

In Matthew 9, a sick woman talks with herself; a common practice amongst people. While it was a connection with Jesus that healed this woman, it was a preliminary interaction the woman had with herself that made the connection with Jesus possible. The woman encourages her soul to believe in the impossible. A golden rule to follow today is don't say anything to yourself you wouldn't say to a child you were coaching.

# SURVIVING FEELINGS WORKSHEET

## 1. Name it (Identification)

_____
_____
_____
_____
_____
_____
_____
_____
_____

## 2. Frame it (Validation)

_____
_____
_____
_____
_____
_____
_____
_____
_____

## 3. Tame it (Regulation)

_____
_____
_____
_____
_____
_____
_____
_____
_____

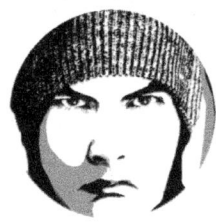

# I FEEL UNTRUSTING TOWARD AUTHORITY

*Be shepherds of God's flock that is among you, watching over them.*
I Peter 5:2

If I hung a sign outside my front door that stated, "Don't spit on the sidewalk", I'd bet that there be more spitting post-sign than pre-sign. Aversion to authority - the urge to rebel against instructions from a higher-up - is a running theme since Adam and Eve. Neuroimaging research indicates that some folks exhibit even higher mistrust towards authority. These studies show changes in two brain regions, the parietal lobule, and the dorsolateral prefrontal cortex, commonly associated with remaining in control. For some people, the need to be in control rather than having others call the shots is biological.

While science has yet to unravel the reasons for this, psychoanalysts suggest that early childhood abuse might be the culprit. In such tragic situations, control is snatched from a child. Therefore, the biological urge to retain control is heightened throughout adulthood. The wounded adult comes to believe that they are only safe when they sit in the cockpit. But, the good news is that the brain can be rewired for those who don't trust so easily,

Scriptures make it clear that shepherds are not just peers among us, but overseers of our souls. Now, you may reason that authority figures have already proven themselves to be hirelings. But, take heed that you don't cancel the real Shepherds whose guidance preserves your soul. It'd be a crying shame to throw away the money in your bank account because there are counterfeit bills in circulation.

# SURVIVING FEELINGS WORKSHEET

### 1. Name it (Identification)

_____
_____
_____
_____
_____
_____
_____
_____
_____

### 2. Frame it (Validation)

_____
_____
_____
_____
_____
_____
_____
_____
_____

### 3. Tame it (Regulation)

_____
_____
_____
_____
_____
_____
_____
_____
_____

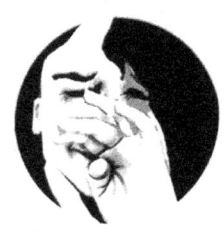

# I FEEL SPIRITUALLY ABUSED

*When ye, therefore, shall see the abomination of desolation, spoken of by Daniel the prophet,*
*erected in the holy place, flee.*

Matthew 24:15

I once fed my dog with the same bowl I filled with motor oil without cleaning it out (a long story). The hound glared up at me disgusted like I played a cruel joke on him. "How could you desecrate the sacred bowl from which I eat?", he mused. Spiritual abuse, the psychological manipulation that happens under the guise of God, bears the same effects on its victims. Folks enter the sanctuary for nourishment but instead find punishment. Like my dog, you might find the places where you eat soiled with fear-tactics, guilt trips, and other manipulative poisons.

Spiritual abuse is when someone overpowers you by using God as a trump card to get what they want. Qualitative studies (research by way of interviews) reveal that spiritual abuse typically includes the following characteristics - using the scriptures to manipulate someone into fulfilling a personal agenda rather than true kingdom business, employing guilt trips or fear tactics rather than love, and ostracizing those who dissent from the flock.

Of course, Matthew 24:15 speaks in a futuristic tone of the Anti-Christ who will defile the holy place with his despicable image. Yet we are told that the spirit of Anti-Christ is not restricted to a person in the future but resides with us in the present. May I submit to you that anytime someone uses Jesus' name or the Word of God to manipulate you, they are operating in an anti-Christ spirit that "desecrates the holy place"? Ultimately, Anti-Christ influences people to abandon religion and become hostile toward Christ. Victims of spiritual abuse, flee from such people. Also, note that the true altar is not erected in a house but established with your heart; you are the temple of God. No one has access to it without your permission. Carry around space inside of your heart reserved for the presence of God alone.

# SURVIVING FEELINGS WORKSHEET

## 1. Name it (Identification)

_____
_____
_____
_____
_____
_____
_____
_____
_____
_____

## 2. Frame it (Validation)

_____
_____
_____
_____
_____
_____
_____
_____
_____
_____

## 3. Tame it (Regulation)

_____
_____
_____
_____
_____
_____
_____
_____
_____
_____

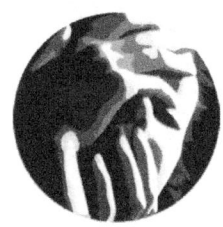

# I FEEL PULLED INTO SOMETHING

*While Joshua was near Jericho, he raised his eyes and saw one who stood facing him, drawn sword in hand. Joshua went up to him and asked, "Are you one of us or one of our enemies?" He replied, "Neither. I am the commander of the Lord's army."*

Joshua 5:13

A fire with a couple of embers eventually dies out. Additional wood keeps the flames burning and sometimes scorching into a conflagration. Likewise, most conflicts between two people, after some time, calm down with a cease-fire. However, battles escalate into long-standing wars when third parties get deeply involved and feel the need to take sides. Are you that third party? Behind the scenes of every massive conflict between parents and children, church families, siblings, and ex-lovers are typically more trouble-makers than peacemakers.

What motivates people to take sides? According to the research of Hogg and Adelman, you often take sides to gain approval or acceptance from the individuals you lock arms with. Perhaps you want that person to like you or notice your loyalty. But when you take sides, you fuel the flames of a feud that was just about to die out. Too many embers keeps the fire burning.

In Joshua 5, Joshua elicits an angel of God to join his army. "Take sides with me", he's saying. It doesn't make it any easier when those at war insist on you choosing sides. But, being a stalwart representative of God himself, the angel refuses to take sides. Instead, he calls himself "commander". Rest assured, when God shows up, He doesn't come as an ally to help you further your petty agenda. Instead, He arrives as an authority to call the shots. He doesn't show up to take sides, but to take over. Likewise, the truest friends in your life aren't interested in enabling your destructive plans. Instead, they show up as conduits to bring about the will of God. Blessed are the peacemakers, not the troublemakers, for they shall be called sons and daughters of God.

---

Uncertainty–Identity Theory (Journal of Social Issues, Hogg and Adelman, 2013)

# SURVIVING FEELINGS WORKSHEET

## 1. Name it (Identification)

_____
_____
_____
_____
_____
_____
_____
_____
_____
_____

## 2. Frame it (Validation)

_____
_____
_____
_____
_____
_____
_____
_____
_____

## 3. Tame it (Regulation)

_____
_____
_____
_____
_____
_____
_____
_____
_____

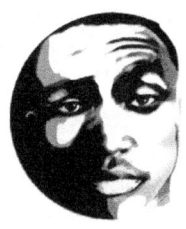

# I FEEL COLD

*Don't let kindness and truth leave you. Bind them around your neck.*
*Write them on the tablet of your heart.*
Proverbs 3:3

Sometimes, the older you get, the colder you get. Overuse of the hands from tilling the ground or shoveling ditches results in callouses. What happens to the hands also happens to the heart; emotions dry up after shedding too many tears. Compassion fatigue is the clinical term used to describe people whose empathy was exchanged for apathy. Such an empathy deficit is the real pandemic of our day.

Chronic exposure to suffering weakens our compassion response. For example, in 2014, a mere $100,000 was raised in six months by the American Red Cross for the loss of 3400 lives from the Ebola outbreak. The general public was inundated with images of the suffering, which inadvertently immobilized their compassion. On the other hand, Harvard raised over $1.2 in less than a month for one underprivileged child to go to college. Harvard kept their campaign simple with a picture of the boy's face and their plea. Whack-job Stalin knew what he was talking about when he said, "The death of one is a tragedy. The death of millions is just a statistic."

King Solomon weaves together two virtues that easily elude us - kindness and truth. No coincidence that he forms this pair because the loss of one (truth) leads to the vanishing of the other (kindness). For instance, we tell ourselves two lies when confronted by a need - Lie #1 "Someone else will take care of it" and Lie #2, "Some other time, I'll help". Next time you walk by someone in need, ask yourself two questions when debating whether you should help - "If not you, then who? If not now, then when?"

# SURVIVING FEELINGS WORKSHEET

## 1. Name it (Identification)

_____
_____
_____
_____
_____
_____
_____
_____
_____

## 2. Frame it (Validation)

_____
_____
_____
_____
_____
_____
_____
_____
_____

## 3. Tame it (Regulation)

_____
_____
_____
_____
_____
_____
_____
_____

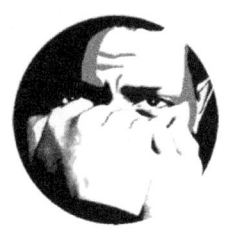

# I FEEL THREATENED

*So Jezebel sent a messenger to Elijah to say, "May the gods deal with me,*
*be it ever so severely if by this time tomorrow I do not make your life like that of one of them."*
I Kings 19:1

At 6 years old, puny me took cover in my bedroom from a brawny kid in the playground who threatened to pulverize my face. Minutes later, mommy and aunty lugged me into that jungle gym, kicking and screaming, to square off with my tormentor. To my astonishment, I caught a peripheral glimpse of that bully bolt back into his building as he noticed me come out. That Saturday morning back in the early 1980s, I swallowed a jagged but invaluable lesson that served me well over the next four decades - Call your bully's bluff and you'll discover their yappers are bigger than their fists.

More often than not, a threat is more fatal in our minds than what it truly is in our midst. Cole and colleagues (2013) demonstrated through a study on the cognitive effects of a threat that fear distorts perception. In the study, participants guesstimated that a tarantula was significantly closer in proximity than a cup when both objects were relatively the same distance. Given the fact that the participants were terrified of the spider, they supposed it was more imminent than it was. When General Patton was asked if he ever felt fear during the war, he replied, "Of course I did. I just never took counsel from my fears." Your fears are the worst advisors so don't pay much attention to what they say.

Regarding the mentioned passage, why does Jezebel feel the need to send Elijah a message? Why not just strike at a moment when he least expects it? Usually, legit opponents don't warn you about what they're gonna do; they just do it. The threat alone is often a red flag that you are dealing with a hoax. Sadly, Elijah ditches his post (probably Jezebel's only goal) all because of a mere threat. Until he learns the lesson I learned in that playground, Jezebel wins. Bullies only hang out in a coward's backyard.

---

*Affective Signals of Threat Increase Perceived Proximity (Sage, Cole et al., 2013)*

# SURVIVING FEELINGS WORKSHEET

## 1. Name it (Identification)

_____

_____

_____

_____

_____

_____

_____

_____

## 2. Frame it (Validation)

_____

_____

_____

_____

_____

_____

_____

_____

## 3. Tame it (Regulation)

_____

_____

_____

_____

_____

_____

_____

_____

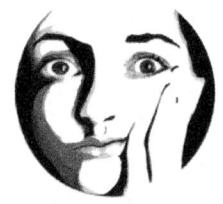

# I FEEL MISUNDERSTOOD

*(Satan is) the prince of the air...* Ephesians 2:2

I once shipped my 28-year-old daughter, who lives in New Orleans, a package that didn't arrive in the same manner I sent it. If Ashley didn't know me better, she would have been insulted by the bag of Catanzaro wine biscuits drenched with marinara sauce. Something unintended occurred between the port of delivery to the point of reception. Have you ever sent a message to someone (via text, email, or even face to face) that wasn't received in the same manner in which you sent it? Suddenly, a rift in the relationship exists because of unintended phenomena between the port of delivery and the point of reception. You think to yourself, "that's not how I meant it (a.k.a., sent it)." Why is it so easy to misunderstand each other?

First is the psychological view. Misunderstandings are probable because of what's known as "the illusion of transparency". This theory asserts that we presume that what we think and feel is more transparent than what it truly is. God, I've been guilty of this many times! We mistakenly assume that folks recognize our mental state more than they do. Stanford University conducted an experiment whereby a participant tapped the well-known "happy birthday" tune with her fingers before an audience. The participant predicted that 50% of the audience knew the tapped tune, but only 3% did! (Newton, 2015). Misunderstandings also happen because of "confirmation bias". We get an idea stuck in our heads of who someone is (e.g., "He's so arrogant") and filter everything they say and do through that preconceived perception. Chances are, you will find whatever you're looking for in someone.

More importantly, the spiritual view. Imagine a 3rd party lingering within the atmosphere between you and the people you talk with. Imagine a 3rd party who's an instigator that insists upon distorting every message you communicate. Imagine a 3rd party who's been granted dominion over the "air(waves)". What you just imagined is real. Ephesians 2:2 describes the enemy of our souls as "the prince of the air". If you value your relationships with people, take the time to "clear the air" on what you said. Continually clearing the air is the only way to ensure that the prince of the air doesn't become king of the air.

---

Happy Birthday Tune Tapped (Stanford University, Newton, 1990)

# SURVIVING FEELINGS WORKSHEET

## 1. Name it (Identification)

_____
_____
_____
_____
_____
_____
_____
_____
_____

## 2. Frame it (Validation)

_____
_____
_____
_____
_____
_____
_____
_____
_____

## 3. Tame it (Regulation)

_____
_____
_____
_____
_____
_____
_____
_____
_____

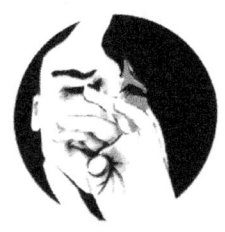

# I FEEL SAD ABOUT A RIFT

*Jesus has given to us the ministry of reconciliation.*  II Corinthians 5:17

Research conducted by Karl Pillemer of Cornell University indicates 1 in 4 adults are estranged from family (Pillemer, 2020). Here are a few suggestions on how to rekindle a relationship.

## Put Your Seat Belt On

Reconcile with the realistic expectation that conflicts are inevitable. When two or more gather, someone is bound to get offended. Jesus in Luke 17:1 promised us that "offenses will come, but woe to the one who brings the offense". Expect to get offended, but don't become offensive when you're offended. Learn to hush when hurt and wait for a better time to address issues.

## Stay In Your Lane

An overwhelming majority of rifts occur because someone doesn't know how to mind their own business.  Reconciliations work when you know your role in someone's life, and you've relegated them to a particular role within your life, and you remain within these lanes. Boundaries must be respected for the relationship to rekindle.

## Look Through the Windshield

The windshield is 37x the size of the rearview mirror which insinuates that where you are headed is far more important than where you've been. Research shows that the common characteristic of unsalvageable relationships is a frequent reference to painful events of the past. Ask yourself the question, "where can we go from here?". Deeply ponder and carefully communicate goals for your relationships such as planning events, activities, and other happenings.

## Trust Your GPS

Driving in uncharted territory can't happen without the higher intelligence of a GPS. Successful reconciliations occur when you realize that you are heading in a direction you've never been before; therefore, you need the HOLY SPIRIT to guide you into all things. Keep in step with the Spirit and His frequent promptings throughout your journey, and you'll have the ride of your life.

---

The Depths of Estrangement (NY Times, Pillemer, 2020)

# SURVIVING FEELINGS WORKSHEET

## 1. Name it (Identification)

_____
_____
_____
_____
_____
_____
_____
_____
_____
_____

## 2. Frame it (Validation)

_____
_____
_____
_____
_____
_____
_____
_____
_____
_____

## 3. Tame it (Regulation)

_____
_____
_____
_____
_____
_____
_____
_____
_____

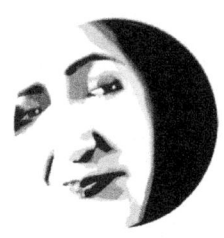

# I FEEL LIKE I'M BEING TALKED ABOUT

*Then the Pharisees went out and began to plot with the Herodians*
*on how they might kill Jesus.*

Mark 3:6

52 minutes - the average time per day devoted to gossip according to a recent study (University of California, 2018). A massive chunk, believe it or not, targets achievers of noteworthy results. Rarely ever do we roast the couch potato living next door; more often than not, we deep-fry the charismatic dude or dame making a blaring difference in our world. "She's only in it for the money" or "He's not the same person at home" are just a few things we say about champions of various causes. So, if you're the subject of such gossip, a motto in Southern politics is worthy of noting, "You know you're standing out front when you're getting kicked in the behind."

A recent study using brain mappings showed that gossip about successful people lights up the striatum. The striatum is the reward center of the brain, inducing feelings of pleasure associated with accomplishing something. Imagine! Gossipers derive a sense of accomplishment in spreading rumors about people who've accomplished something. In the worldview of a gossiper, if you can't make a difference in the world; attack someone who is making a difference and it'll feel equally good.

What's so curious about Mark 3:6 is the union between two groups of people conspiring against Jesus - the Pharisees and the Herodians. On any given day, these two sects hated each other! You'd be hard-pressed to find these fellas chilling at a Jewish deli chomping on bagels and lox. The only thing that would instigate such a gossipy union is someone like Jesus, making a noteworthy difference in the world. If you've been hurt by what you're hearing other people are saying about you, you're in good company. Be not dismayed - it could be a sign you're up to big things! In the words of Oscar Wilde, "You know what's worse than being talked about? Not being talked about." Selah.

---

Social Psychological and Personality Science Journal (University of California, 2018)

# SURVIVING FEELINGS WORKSHEET

## 1. Name it (Identification)

_____

_____

_____

_____

_____

_____

_____

_____

_____

## 2. Frame it (Validation)

_____

_____

_____

_____

_____

_____

_____

_____

_____

## 3. Tame it (Regulation)

_____

_____

_____

_____

_____

_____

_____

_____

_____

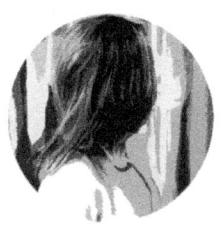

# I FEEL DISSATISFIED

*Those who work their land will have abundant food,*
*but those who chase fantasies have no sense.*

Proverbs 12:11

Presuming that "something else" will make you happy is the great delusion of mankind. Eve had paradise in her midst yet was hoodwinked into believing that "something else" would be even better. Since that cataclysmic moment in the garden, the chase has been on! Such a restlessness causes people to switch careers, relationships, geographies, physical appearances, etc. supposing that "something else" will plug that hole in my soul. The facts are that you won't be happy with what you want until you've found satisfaction in what you have.

Wilson & Gilbert (2005) demonstrated through a study that college students grossly overestimated how happy they'd be if they switched to a more preferred dorm room. Other similar experiments indicated that sports fans miscalculated the degree of ecstasy they'd experience if their favorite team won. These experiments highlight a theory known as Impact Bias, a cognitive glitch whereby we overestimate how happy something else will make us. Our predictors of what will make us smile are broken!

Wise Solomon exposes the lunacy of chasing fantasies in Proverbs 12. Fantasy is defined as something more actual in your mentality than it is in reality. Solomon calls those who seek after something else "senseless". In contrast, he depicts the fruitful man as one who works the land he already owns. Fulfillment comes not from seizing something else...another house, another spouse, another blouse...but from loving the one you're already with.

---

Affective Forecasting (Sage, Wilson and Gilbert, 2005)

# SURVIVING FEELINGS WORKSHEET

## 1. Name it (Identification)

_____
_____
_____
_____
_____
_____
_____
_____
_____
_____

## 2. Frame it (Validation)

_____
_____
_____
_____
_____
_____
_____
_____
_____

## 3. Tame it (Regulation)

_____
_____
_____
_____
_____
_____
_____
_____
_____

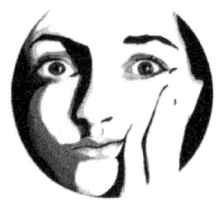

# I FEEL AIMLESS

*Then the LORD replied: "Write down the revelation and*
*make it plain on tablets so that a herald may run with it."*
Habakkuk 2:2

Some folks squander their existence by staring up the steps. "One day, I shall go upstairs", they bloviate about dreams of the future while gazing into the unknown. Months ripen into years, and they're still staring up the steps. Bump into them in the supermarket, and you'll hear them ramble about the same pie-in-the-sky ideas from yesteryear. Others, a scant handful, actually step up the stairs. They regularly make headway on what they purpose to do. For these folks, a narrow gap exists between imagination and implementation. They wake up every morning seeking ways to translate what they're seeing into being. Dreamers stare up the steps, whereas doers step up the stairs.

What distinguishes the dreamer from the doer? A Harvard Business Study discovered that people with written goals are 3x more successful than those who don't write them down. Other research found that writing down your goals makes you 42% more like to achieve them (Gail, 2018). Writing down your goals increases your likelihood of achievement in a few ways - First, it brings accountability. Second, it brings specificity to abstract notions. Warren Buffet described writing as the act of refining his jumbled thoughts. Lastly, it brings order. We are more likely to follow step-by-step sequences than random tasks.

After a few moments of envisioning, the Lord instructs the prophet to write down what he sees. God commands him, "Make the abstract concrete by putting pen to pad." For what reason? So that the herald can run with the vision. A vision without words is a vision without feet. But a vision written down is a plan that's about to go down! Feeling aimless and don't know where to begin? Start by writing down the vision inside of you,

How to Write Down Your Goals (University of California, Matthews, 2018)

# SURVIVING FEELINGS WORKSHEET

1. Name it (Identification)

_____

_____

_____

_____

_____

_____

_____

_____

_____

2. Frame it (Validation)

_____

_____

_____

_____

_____

_____

_____

_____

_____

3. Tame it (Regulation)

_____

_____

_____

_____

_____

_____

_____

_____

_____

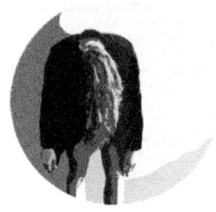

# I FEEL DIRTY

*But if we walk in the light, as He is in the light, we have fellowship one with another, and the*
*blood of Jesus Christ His Son cleanseth us from all sin.*

I John 1:7

Moral transgressions leave us feeling filthy. Glancing at porn, pilfering from the tip jar, duping our neighbor, and betraying our conscience on any level smudges the soul with grime that no antiseptic can expunge. Our divine origin (the fact that we were made in God's image) is like being dressed in a glistening white outfit where stains stand out. Moral filth would have no impact on us if we were made in the likeness of Lucifer, just like stains leave no impression on a charcoal shirt. Being made in God's image, while simultaneously marred by Adam's sin, is like being a slob dressed in a pristine outfit that flaunts all the food we splatter. After we've sinned, we feel dirty only because we were initially made to be holy.

For the reasons stated above, we resort to "purging acts" to sanitize our filth after we've sinned. Behavioral scientists conducted a study where they divided participants into two groups - the first group was asked to reflect upon a recent moral failure whereas the second group (control group) was free to think about anything. After the time of reflection, both groups were offered a gift - a cleansing wipe or a new pencil. Participants who reflected upon moral failures were 3x more likely to choose the cleansing wipe. This study reveals our instinct to purge our moral filth; an instinct that surfaces in a myriad of ways. I've known pedophiles who've donated thousands to charity to scrub their souls of the feeling of filth. And the list goes on. Often, people are so nice only because they are also so nasty.

The Apostle John sheds light on the power of the blood of Christ. Other verses speak of the blood "forgiving" our sins, an objective reality whereby the Almighty Judge exonerates us from a justifiable death sentence. But this verse speaks of the blood "cleansing" our sins, a subjective reality whereby our conscience is scrubbed of all guilt. The truth is, we need cleansing in addition to forgiveness. It's one thing to be forgiven. It's another thing to feel forgiven. Interesting to note that this washing only occurs when we "fellowship with one another". The verse insinuates that the church, the fellowship of the saints, is a spiritual bathhouse where our souls are sanitized individually and collectively.

---

*Study Finds That Washing Eases Guilty Conscience (NY Times, Carey, 2006)*

# SURVIVING FEELINGS WORKSHEET

## 1. Name it (Identification)

_____
_____
_____
_____
_____
_____
_____
_____
_____

## 2. Frame it (Validation)

_____
_____
_____
_____
_____
_____
_____
_____
_____
_____

## 3. Tame it (Regulation)

_____
_____
_____
_____
_____
_____
_____
_____
_____
_____

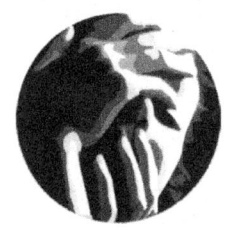

# I FEEL STUCK

*Repent, for the kingdom of heaven is at hand.*

Matthew 3:2

While in Dallas, I ended up on the wrong side of the highway on a road without any U-Turns. I might be a Ph.D. in behavioral science but I'm a dullard with directions. There it was, the church on my left, as I drove passed it with no ability to U-Turn for another 15 miles! Trying to break a habit is much like endeavoring to turn around on one of those peculiar highways in Texas. Once habits are formed, the soul speedily advances towards its object of desire without any grace to about-face.

The golden rule for predicting a person's behavior is to study their narrative. Pay attention to a subject long enough, and you'll cease being surprised. The most reliable forecast for what a subject will do next is what they already did. Even if the subject changes directions, it's typically only a matter of time before they return to their former ways. For instance, documentary research conducted by behavioral scientists on a particular season of "The Biggest Loser" showed that 14 out of 15 contestants who lost dramatic weight put it back on in less than two years. Other studies show that a person who cheats on their spouse is 350% more likely to cheat again than someone who's never cheated. That's not just true about others. We are all on a road with no U-Turns.

Regarding Matthew 3:2, the call to repentance is an opportunity that often comes out of nowhere to U-turn on a road headed over a cliff. You firmly resolve that you're gonna hook up with him alone at his hotel despite the ring on that finger with a vein that shoots directly to the heart. You curl your hair, apply mascara and adorn yourself in the sexiest dress. You responded to his most recent text with an assurance that you'll be there soon. There's no going back now. Just as you turn over the ignition, your heartbeat races fast and you sense an urge to turn back. Of course, you are free to resist that urge but it's available nonetheless. That particular urge is not merely a psychological sensation, but an invitation from God himself. Repentance is not a gloomy word that some preachers have made it, but a supernatural gift that descends from above; a grace to about-face on a road headed to destruction.

# SURVIVING FEELINGS WORKSHEET

### 1. Name it (Identification)

_____

_____

_____

_____

_____

_____

_____

_____

_____

_____

### 2. Frame it (Validation)

_____

_____

_____

_____

_____

_____

_____

_____

_____

### 3. Tame it (Regulation)

_____

_____

_____

_____

_____

_____

_____

_____

_____

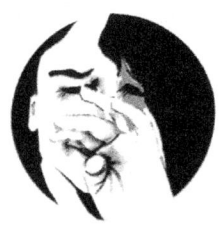

# I FEEL LIKE HURTING MYSELF

*By His stripes, we are healed.*

Isaiah 53:5

Why do people cut themselves? Basic economics teaches us that you can't obtain a product without paying a price. If you're craving a chocolate bar, it's gonna cost you $2.30. You have to pay a price to obtain a product. Oddly enough, this is what drives a self-mutilator to lacerate their body. Daisy, a character in the film GIRL INTERRUPTED, cuts her arms to experience relief (a feeling that any girl trapped in a body sexually violated by their father yearns to experience). Daisy is paying a price for a product she desires. Allow me to explain how this works...

Behavioral scientists conceptualized a theory known as Pain Offset Relief in their attempt to understand self-masochism. Behavioral scientists learned via experiments that people cut themselves to experience the short, but intense, period of euphoria that happens after they stop cutting. Dopamine (pleasure) levels are higher after being inflicted with pain than the state of mind before the cutting. In short, cutters aren't as crazy as they seem. Cutters are merely doing the same math as every consumer who empties their pocket for a caramel Twix. They are paying a price to obtain the desired product.

We are economical creatures who presume a price should be paid for every product. The Old Testament's sacrificial system reflects our instinctual need to slaughter something precious to receive something valuable. In Isaiah 53:5, God presents healing that wasn't free by any means. No truly good thing is free or offered at a wholesale rate. The verse alludes to the healing of our souls purchased at the cross of Jesus Christ. The essence of the gospel is that by accepting what Christ did for us, we are heirs to all of the goods of heaven (peace, love, joy) without having to lacerate ourselves. Cutters, take heed - the price has already been paid. Your only due service is to care for the temple that houses the gift of Christ.

The Nature of Pain Offset Relief (Sage, Franklin et al., 2013)

# SURVIVING FEELINGS WORKSHEET

1. Name it (Identification)

_____
_____
_____
_____
_____
_____
_____
_____
_____
_____

2. Frame it (Validation)

_____
_____
_____
_____
_____
_____
_____
_____
_____
_____

3. Tame it (Regulation)

_____
_____
_____
_____
_____
_____
_____
_____
_____
_____

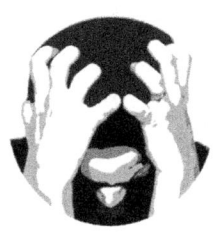

# I FEEL GUILTY

*But beloved, we are persuaded better things for you, things that accompany your salvation.*

Hebrews 6:9

Motor Week published a recent article about cheap gas having long-term effects on its engine. Guilt trips are much like cheap gas; they mobilize people for short spurts but impede motivation over the long haul. In my earlier years of pastoring, the prayer meetings on Tuesday nights were crammed after I badgered the people about being carnal for not praying enough in the Sunday sermon. Cheap gas mobilized them from their Lazy-boy to the altars...at least for that Tuesday. The prayer meeting was jammed. But, the following week's prayer meeting was usually empty. What I was too naive to realize was that guilt trips undermine long-term motivation by depicting prayer as a chore rather than something to adore.

Columbia University conducted a study on the impact of guilt trips versus a booster shot of pride in motivating people. Participants in Group 1 were asked to mull over their lack of concern for the environment, inducing inevitable feelings of guilt. Participants in Group 2 were requested to reflect upon their concern for the environment, and how good it would feel to take care of what belongs to them. After the self-reflective activity, Group 1 revealed substantially less willingness in adopting long-term shopping and traveling modifications that would improve the environment than Group 2.

Note the booster shot of confidence that the writer of Hebrews injects into a backslidden church in verse 6:9, "But beloved, we are persuaded better things for you...". Through such language, the writer draws out the best in them rather than accentuating the worst in them. This approach inspires an internal change by tapping into the desire to want to be better, a yearning that God places inside every one of His reborn children. Internal change is much better than imposed change. Internal change is like an egg hatching from within; life emerges. Imposed change (via guilt trips) is like an egg cracked from without; dead yolk leaks out. Hatched eggs are more enlivening than cracked eggs. Let change happen from within rather than being imposed from without.

The Influence of Anticipated Pride and Guilt (Plos One, Schnieder et al., 2017)

# SURVIVING FEELINGS WORKSHEET

## 1. Name it (Identification)

_____
_____
_____
_____
_____
_____
_____
_____
_____

## 2. Frame it (Validation)

_____
_____
_____
_____
_____
_____
_____
_____
_____

## 3. Tame it (Regulation)

_____
_____
_____
_____
_____
_____
_____
_____
_____

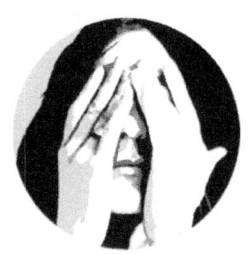

# I FEEL TORN

*We have peace with God through our Lord Jesus Christ.*

Romans 5:1

Oh, such angst in trying to assemble pieces of a puzzle that won't fit together! Just the mere sight of those seemingly unrelated cardboard cutouts, scattered across your kitchen table, drives you mad if you stare at them too long. Some of our minds are like that puzzle - irreconcilable pieces that cause inner turmoil. For instance, you harbor conflicting views of yourself. There's one piece of yourself you like way too much; a vanity that shows itself through bragging and boasting. But then, there's this other piece of yourself you hate; a self-loathing that reveals itself through masochistic activities. Many emotional troubles arise from a psyche in pieces.

Splitting is a psychological term to describe the psyche that cannot reconcile opposing realities much like a person that can't put pieces of a puzzle together. Splitters perceive everything in terms of good or evil, black or white. Splitters either love and adore you, or loath and abhor you. You are either on their greatest hits list, or you are on their hit list. You rank as a hero one second, and a zero the next. This is equally true of how splitters feel about themselves. Splitters defend themselves as the sacrificial martyr of the family today, then verbally berate themselves as an awful person tomorrow. There's no in-between because their minds cannot reconcile variant pieces into one puzzle (Facts are, we are all mixed bags but the splitting psyche cannot accept that. Splitters have no peace because their psyche is in pieces).

Shalom is the Hebrew term of Romans 5:1, a word that means the peace that results from being properly integrated or made whole. Shalom, in its simplest definition, means "made whole". Ah, that blissful relief you experience when the puzzle is finally put together! But Shalom is not just when your psyche is integrated within itself. First and foremost, Shalom is your psyche being reconciled with God! Sin has separated us from our maker. So, you want the peace of God (less splitting), make peace with God. You cannot experience the peace of God until you've made peace with God. You'll be made whole within yourself when you've been made one with Him. And being in peace is so much better than being in pieces.

# SURVIVING FEELINGS WORKSHEET

1. Name it (Identification)

_____

_____

_____

_____

_____

_____

_____

_____

2. Frame it (Validation)

_____

_____

_____

_____

_____

_____

_____

3. Tame it (Regulation)

_____

_____

_____

_____

_____

_____

_____

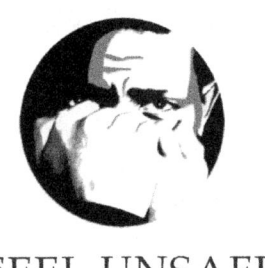

# I FEEL UNSAFE

*He prepares a table before me in the presence of my enemies.*

Psalm 23

Bolted doors, a 35mm under your pillow, and a house in the hills will NOT fully satiate your need for safety. Moving out of Boston or NYC into rural America won't make you feel as secure as you suppose. Instead, these security measures reinforce the fact that you live in a capricious world. Soon, you'll toss and turn throughout the night wondering, "If I'm safe, then why do I need a gun?" The adage is true - you can run, but you can't hide. If safety cannot be found in a loaded weapon or a remote location, what will make me feel secure?

Abraham Maslow theorized that you'll never manifest your potential until you feel safe. Maslow's model suggested that the need to feel safe is pivotal for success on all avenues of life. Since 1946, Maslow's theory has been demonstrated through countless studies where participants do better when they feel safe. Students perform better on tests, adults with addictions stay sober longer and employees achieve higher benchmarks when they feel safe. Once again, if safety is so paramount, what will make me feel secure?

Oddly enough, in Psalm 23, the songwriter does not describe safety as the distance from danger. The psalmist doesn't say, "He prepares a table before me far from my enemies". Instead, he depicts the safe place as being close to whatever threatens you with his phrase, "...in the presence of my enemies". The formula for safety is when the presence of God mightily presides over wherever danger closely resides. You don't feel truly covered by an umbrella until the rains come down hard, you don't feel protected by an anchor until the waves rage and you won't feel sheltered by God until danger approaches. Safety is when God shows up amidst a near and present danger.

# SURVIVING FEELINGS WORKSHEET

## 1. Name it (Identification)

_____
_____
_____
_____
_____
_____
_____
_____
_____
_____

## 2. Frame it (Validation)

_____
_____
_____
_____
_____
_____
_____
_____
_____

## 3. Tame it (Regulation)

_____
_____
_____
_____
_____
_____
_____
_____
_____

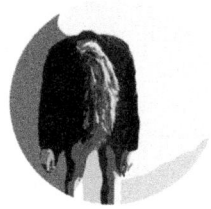

# I FEEL FRUITLESS/UNPRODUCTIVE

*When Jesus reached the tree, he found nothing but leaves. He said to the tree,*

*"May no one ever eat fruit from you again."*

Mark 11:13

"Don't be a quitter!" undoubtedly ranks on Family Feud as the single most repetitious mantra recited by parents to their children. Who could ever argue with such a winner's logic that propelled guys like Churchill to advance onward during the darkest hours? However, occasions arise when good advice morphs into bad counsel like fresh bread turning stale. Consider that the conviction of never quitting is what keeps a man or woman stuck in an abusive relationship or the CEO of a company remaining at the helm of a failing corporation. The most successful people recall at least 1 example from the journey where they had to cut losses.

Why is it so hard to quit? Behavioral scientists propose a theory to this question based on multiple case studies known as the "justification of effort theory". The justification of effort theory asserts that we find it difficult to quit because it invalidates the amount of time and energy we invested into something. According to this theory, we have to justify our previous investments to reduce cognitive dissonance (inner turmoil) so we stay longer than we should. For instance, a woman might reason, "How could I leave him now after I've spent so much time and energy believing for him to change?" Walking away from the relationship is too difficult because it makes her feel like she wasted a decade of her life. An executive might feel the same way about his precious company.

Jesus certainly knew when it was time to cut losses. In Mark 11:13, Jesus finds a beloved fig tree that was planted and nurtured by someone. The Savior discovers a tree that He co-labored with the Father in designing during the Genesis creation account. Yet, he curses it into death. He calls it "quits" on sustaining the tree's life. Why? According to bible commentator William Barclay, fig trees are one of the few plants that bear fruit before leaves. The fact that the tree is bearing leaves but not fruit means it's not producing the expected results. Kenny Rogers once penned a wise lyric, "you gotta know when to hold 'em and you gotta know when to fold 'em". Perhaps it's time to curse some fig-less trees today.

# SURVIVING FEELINGS WORKSHEET

## 1. Name it (Identification)

_____

_____

_____

_____

_____

_____

_____

_____

_____

## 2. Frame it (Validation)

_____

_____

_____

_____

_____

_____

_____

_____

_____

## 3. Tame it (Regulation)

_____

_____

_____

_____

_____

_____

_____

_____

_____

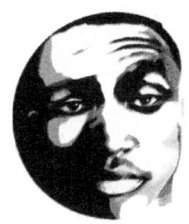

# I FEEL LIFELESS

*If the same spirit that rose Jesus from the dead dwells in you,*
*that spirit will bring life to your mortal body.*

Romans 8:11

In a relatively short time, I officiated the funerals of 13 relatives and friends whom I loved dearly; the hardest being a 29-year-old spiritual daughter who was 8 months pregnant at her passing. I endured a brutal divorce after being married for 19 years. I survived 2 heart attacks, the 2nd being the widow-maker that kills 83% of its quarry. I resigned from a 16-year career of pastoring. I experienced betrayal at deep levels. I've been lied about by people who mattered. I'll spare you the ugly details of other private ordeals that'd make you cringe. All of these graves brought me down, but none of these graves kept me down. What graves did you ascend from over the last few years? I'm sure you have your own comeback story. Selah.

The Holmes-Rahe Life Stress Inventory measures the traumatic impact of life events upon a person's psyche. The inventory assigns a numerical value to each life event (a value that derives from statistical analysis of people who experienced mental breakdowns as a result of the event). I personally withstood 5 of the top 10 events listed within the inventory. Such a reality says I should be locked away within a rubber room, garbed in a straight jacket, while the nurse wipes the drool from my chin as I mumble "papa". Instead, I sit here dressed in my right mind. How do I explain such resilience?

The facts are that I'm a highly sensitive person. I'm the fella who absorbs equally as much as I observe, meaning that I emotionally take in my circumstances. In no way, shape, or form can I attribute my comebacks to a mentally tough demeanor. I'm fragile. Instead, I accredit my ascension to the power described in Romans 8. The Apostle Paul says that we believers come back from every setback for one simple reason - not because of a resilient personality but because of the resurrection reality. If Jesus walked out of the grave, then it stands to reason that His followers are walking out too. Ain't no grave gonna hold my body down.

# SURVIVING FEELINGS WORKSHEET

## 1. Name it (Identification)

_____
_____
_____
_____
_____
_____
_____
_____
_____

## 2. Frame it (Validation)

_____
_____
_____
_____
_____
_____
_____
_____
_____

## 3. Tame it (Regulation)

_____
_____
_____
_____
_____
_____
_____
_____
_____

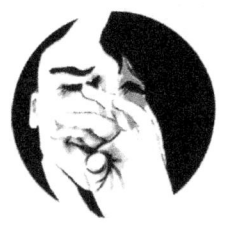

# I FEEL UNLOVABLE

*And the Lord brought the woman to the man.*
Genesis 2:22

My picker is broken. If a choice had to be made between the delicious and the nutritious, I almost always select the delicious over the nutritious. Stand behind me in a buffet line, and you'll see 98.7% of my plate crammed with barbecue ribs, baked mac and cheese, crispy French fries, and a half of a broccoli leaf (smothered in cheddar cheese). Sadly enough, this broken "picker" doesn't just stop with food....it applies to every domain of life apart from the guidance of God.

I don't need you to Amen me. I already know, based on lots of anecdotal evidence, scientific studies, and biblical data, that your picker is broken too. For instance, Forestall (2018) conducted a study on babies shortly after their birth. Results indicated that babies prefer sweet, unhealthy tastes over the bitterness of green foods. If a child prefers healthy foods at a later age, it means that caretakers conditioned their palates for nutritious eating. From the womb, we arrive on planet earth with a broken picker. As they say in Italian, Il mioraccoglitore è rotto!e

In Genesis 2:22, the first person that Eve sees when she emerges from the man's rib is God. She finds God who leads her to the man whose hidden in Him. Single people, you should be so hidden in God that your mate must seek Him to locate you. Furthermore, Adam has no choice in selecting his bride. There's no conversation whereby God inquires, "So Adam, what do you like in a woman?" Instead, God escorts the woman to the man. Of course, his jaw drops at her appearance ("this alas is bone of my bones, flesh of my flesh!"). The best marriages are arranged marriages; not coordinated by the cupids of this earth but facilitated by God himself. Let Him do the picking.

---

Flavor Perception and Preference Development (Annals of Nutrition, Forestell, 2017)

# SURVIVING FEELINGS WORKSHEET

## 1. Name it (Identification)

_____

_____

_____

_____

_____

_____

_____

_____

_____

## 2. Frame it (Validation)

_____

_____

_____

_____

_____

_____

_____

_____

_____

_____

## 3. Tame it (Regulation)

_____

_____

_____

_____

_____

_____

_____

_____

_____

_____

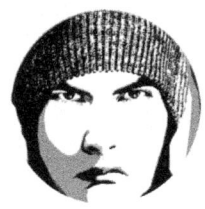

# I FEEL DEJECTED

*...while we wait for the blessed hope, the appearing of the glory*
*our great God and Savior Jesus Christ.*

Titus 2:13

"Someday..." is the preface of many thoughts whenever we're fearful or tearful. Someday, I will be plucked out of this degrading circumstance. Someday, I will be pretzeled with a loving companion under these lonely sheets. Someday, I will receive the justice withheld from me by dumb mortals with gavels. When I interviewed David Berkowitz, a.k.a the Son of Sam, I learned that he dreamt from 4-years old onward of being rescued by his biological father, Joseph Kleinman; a man whom he never met. Berkowitz suffered from what I believe to be a hybrid of mental psychosis (more than likely, schizophrenia) and true demonic possession. Under such duress as a child into adolescence, he religiously fantasized about being rescued. Someday, daddy will save me. Like Berkowitz, we all possess hidden rescue wishes.

The Flight Instinct is not something we learn from watching Marvel flicks but a predisposition from birth. Studies show that infants become fidgety whenever uncomfortable as their way of saying, "Get me out of this!" (Einspieler et al., 2005). The research on childhood abuse reveals a common habit amongst scandalized children to fantasize about being liberated (Somer et al., 2020). Such an instinct bursts out of us all throughout life. Perhaps this inclination was hardwired into us by God to insinuate the reality of His second coming. Desires alone often suggest the reality of something. In the words of CS Lewis, "A duckling yearns to swim because there is such a thing as water". In the same way, we yearn to be rescued because there is such a thing as the Rescuer.

The Greek term that the Apostle Paul applies to describe the Second Coming in Titus 2:13 is "epiphania". The term alludes to the ascension of a great emperor during a dark time. "Epiphania" appeals to our need to be rescued from every form of oppression. For the believer, the second coming of Christ is our ticket out of a nightmare into a blissful reality (For the unbeliever, well, that warrants a more dreadful post)). Believers, we are all fidgety babies wanting and waiting to be scooped up by the arms of our Heavenly Father.

The General Movement Assessment (Frontiers in Psychology, Einspieler, 2016)
Childhood Trauma and Maladaptive Daydreaming (Trauma Dissociation, Somer et al., 2021)

# SURVIVING FEELINGS WORKSHEET

## 1. Name it (Identification)

_____
_____
_____
_____
_____
_____
_____
_____
_____
_____

## 2. Frame it (Validation)

_____
_____
_____
_____
_____
_____
_____
_____
_____
_____

## 3. Tame it (Regulation)

_____
_____
_____
_____
_____
_____
_____
_____
_____
_____

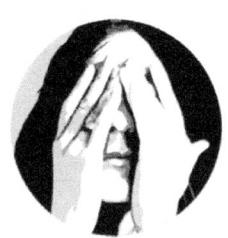

# I FEEL DEPRESSED

Depression is a blanket term we throw on ourselves when we're not sure what's wrong with us. I'm fully persuaded that obscurity alone deepens the melancholy. Hence, Proverbs tells us, "With all thy getting, get understanding". Here's what lies underneath the blanket of depression...

### Fear-Based

The prophet Elijah's depression is set off by Jezebel's threat to kill him in I Kings 19. This threat instigates his depressive cycle. Likewise, some folks are depressed because they're living under the threat of losing their life or something they cherish.

### Guilt-Based

After David sinned with Bathsheba, he said in Psalm 31, "When I kept silent about my sin, my bones wasted away while my soul groaned all day long". Likewise, some folk's depression is the result of harboring guilt over past sins.

### Grief-Based

After losing his children and livelihood, Job says in Job 30:16, "My life seeps away. Depression haunts my days." Likewise, some folks are depressed because of losses.

### Socially-Based

I'm not certain how Adam was behaving in Genesis 2:18. But, his behaviors were so maladjusted that God said, "It's not good for man to be alone." Isolation itself is a basis for all sorts of neurotic and psychotic behaviors.

### Chemically-Based

Psalm 34:19 says, "Many are the afflictions of the righteous but the Lord will deliver him from them all". The Hebrew term for afflicted means a "sick or sad heart". The term refers to a malady of our biology. Facts are our biology is comprised of certain chemicals that keep us well - Dopamine, Seratonin, etc. A deficiency within these areas results in a sad heart.

# SURVIVING FEELINGS WORKSHEET

### 1. Name it (Identification)

_____

_____

_____

_____

_____

_____

_____

_____

_____

### 2. Frame it (Validation)

_____

_____

_____

_____

_____

_____

_____

_____

_____

### 3. Tame it (Regulation)

_____

_____

_____

_____

_____

_____

_____

_____

_____

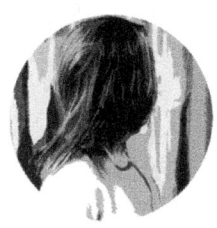

# I FEEL OFFENDED

*If you are without chastening, you are illegitimate and not sons.*

Hebrews 12:8

My spiritual father, Pasco Manzo, hired me in early 2004 as a full-time associate a few years after publicly rebuking me from the pulpit. Unlike many church-goers I knew post-rebuke, I returned every Sunday with an open heart, a marked-up Bible, and a muted tongue. Years later, my pastor informed me that I was the man for the job because I knew how to "take my medicine". I learned that chastening was integral to the process of crawling from bad to good and leaping from good to great. Might sound harsh to the faint-hearted, but I knew my pastor loved me. Shakespeare's Hamlet said it right when he uttered, "the man was cruel to be kind".

Even the secular world recognizes the value of chastening. College ballers would never qualify for the NBA without years of a mentor drilling them. Mueller & Dweck (1998) conducted an experiment amongst grade-school kids that showed constructive feedback is superior to shallow praise. In the study, recipients of shallow praise lacked the resilience to recover after a mistake. But, those subjected to critique brushed themselves off easier. Chosen ones are in dire need of someone to chasten them. God designed the human body so that it's physically awkward to kick yourself in the butt. You need someone else's foot to break through your barriers.

Hebrews 12 takes this concept of chastening to the next level (Of course, true chastening is not abusive but redemptive. The contrast warrants another in-depth post). The verse teaches that our response to chastening not only affects our productivity but reflects our identity. Without mincing words, the writer of Hebrews states that the veracity of sonship is tested by chastening. Pastors, if you lovingly chasten someone and they return, they are a son. If you lovingly chasten someone and they disappear (because of offense), they are a bastard. Sadly, the church has too many bastards and not enough sons. May you be a son or daughter that can handle correction without offense.

---

Praise for Intelligence Can Undermine Children's Motivation (Journal of Personality, Mueller et al., 1998)

# SURVIVING FEELINGS WORKSHEET

## 1. Name it (Identification)

_____

_____

_____

_____

_____

_____

_____

_____

_____

_____

## 2. Frame it (Validation)

_____

_____

_____

_____

_____

_____

_____

_____

_____

## 3. Tame it (Regulation)

_____

_____

_____

_____

_____

_____

_____

_____

_____

_____

Made in the USA
Middletown, DE
07 October 2022

12229411R00084